Street Science

Urban and Industrial Environments

Series editor: Robert Gottlieb, Henry R. Luce Professor of Urban and Environmental Policy, Occidental College

Street Science

Community Knowledge and Environmental Health Justice

Jason Corburn

The MIT Press
Cambridge, Massachusetts
London, England

MIT Press books may be purchased at special quantity discounts for business or sales promotional use. For information, please email special_sales@mitpress.mit.edu or write to Special Sales Department, The MIT Press, 55 Hayward Street, Cambridge, MA 02142.

This book was set in Sabon by Binghamton Valley Composition, LLC
Printed and bound in the United States of America.

Library of Congress Cataloging-in-Publication Data

Corburn, Jason.
Street science : community knowledge and environmental health justice / Jason Corburn.
    p.   cm. — (Urban and industrial environments)
Includes bibliographical references and index.
ISBN 978-0-262-03333-6 (hc. alk. paper) — ISBN 978-0-262-53272-3 (pbk. : alk. paper)
1. Environmental health—Public opinion.   2. Environmental health—Citizen participation.   3. Environmental policy—Citizen participation.
4. Environmental justice.   5. Community.   I. Title.   II. Series.
RA565.C67   2005
362.196'98—dc22   2005047153

Printed on Recycled Paper.

10   9   8   7   6   5

The Mayor   As usual, you employ violent expressions in your report. You say, amongst other things, that what we offer visitors in our Baths is a permanent supply of poison.

Dr. Stockmann   Well, can you describe it any other way, Peter? I tell you—whether you drink it or bathe in it—the water is poison! And this we offer to the poor sick folk who come here in good faith and pay us at an exorbitant rate expecting to be cured!

The Mayor   Believe me, the public has no need of new ideas; it's better off without them. The public is best served by the good, old established ideas it already has.

Dr. Stockmann   This is too much! I, a doctor, a man of science, have no right to—!

The Mayor   But this is not purely a scientific matter; there are other questions involved—technical and economic questions.

Dr. Stockmann   But the source is poisoned, man! Are you mad? Do you want the town to grow rich by selling filth and poison? The whole of our flourishing municipal life derives its sustenance from a lie!

The Mayor   That's worse than nonsense—it's downright libelous! The man who can throw out such offensive insinuations about his native town must be an enemy to our community.

—Henrick Ibsen, "An Enemy of the People" (1882)

I understand the vocation of the intellectual as trying to turn easy answers into critical questions and putting those critical questions to people with power. The quest for truth, the quest for the good, the quest for the beautiful all require us to let suffering speak, let victims be visible and let social misery be put on the agenda of those with power. So to me, pursuing the life of the mind is inextricably linked with the struggle of those who have been dehumanized on the margins of society.

—Cornell West (1999)

Contents

Acknowledgments

This book would not have been possible with out the help and coopera-tion of a number of folks, all of whom I owe a great debt of gratitude. Colleagues at MIT helped me conceive the project as my doctoral disser-tation, including Larry Susskind, David Laws, and Martin Rein. Both John Forester of Cornell and Sheila Jasanoff of Harvard were generous with their time, sat on my dissertation committee, and offered critical and insightful comments. Of course, this book would not have been pos-sible without the activists in Williamsburg sharing their stories with me, especially: Analia Penachasdeh, John Fleming, Cecila Iglesias Garden, Luis Garden-Acosta, Robert Ledogar, Samara Swanston, Rabbi David Neiderman, Kristina Lawson, and Renata Joblonski. Dan Kass, Eva Hanhardt, Gail Suchman, and Joe Ketas also offered their time gener-ously, allowed me to probe the details of their work, and provided me with unlimited access to useful documents. Torri Estrada provided cru-cial insights on the environmental justice movement. David Kotelchuck of Hunter has been a mentor and supported me through the end stages of the project. Mindy Fullilove and Nick Freudenberg offered editorial comments and pushed me to emphasize power inequalities and see the big picture.

Much of the writing took place in 2000 and 2001 during a dissertation fellowship from the Harvard Law School, Program on Negotiation. I also was able to focus on the book after receiving a Robert Wood Johnson Health and Society Scholar postdoctorate fellowship in 2003.

Most important, the inspiration and support for this project has come from Judea and Azure, my soul mates and best friends.

Introduction

A dust cloud from the rubble of the former World Trade Center in lower Manhattan was swirling overhead when I entered a public meeting about local air quality on October 5, 2001. Entering the meeting, I overheard a middle-aged woman who lives in nearby Battery Park City ask her anxious-looking friend: "How can two 100-story buildings disintegrate into thin air—given all the things in those buildings that were never meant to disappear into the air—and that air be perfectly safe to breathe?" Almost on queue, Joel A. Miele Sr., the city's commissioner of the Department of Environmental Protection, came over the microphone and insisted that the air quality, while it might cause nagging discomfort, "is not a health problem. It is human nature," he continued, "to be worried and skeptical, but you can rest assured there is no danger from breathing the air."

The woman next to me was not buying it: "I don't trust them for a minute. We feel physically sick when we stay there, sore throats, burning eyes, rashes." Mary Mears, a spokeswoman for the U.S. Environmental Protection Agency (EPA) got up to calm the uneasiness in the crowd: "You can see the dust, you can taste the dust, you can smell the smoke," she said. "I can understand why people are not convinced based on the evidence they see. By the time I get to work I feel like I was licking the sidewalk."

The EPA and the city's Department of Health had tested the air and tests revealed that only a few samples of heavy metals, asbestos, and other pollutants exceeded health safety levels; of 442 air samples the EPA analyzed for asbestos, only 27 exceeded safety levels (Saulny and Reukin 2001). "The chances of being exposed now are miniscule," noted commissioner Miele.

Walking out of the meeting, I caught up with the woman who had been sitting next to me. I asked whether the meeting had reassured her. She commented:

What did they tell us? Essentially, that after they study the effects of the air on a variety of populations for the next few years they'd have lots of interesting data to report. They thoughtfully described their studies for us, although I noted the lack of research on immune system disorders, the type of problem I have. Their comments on stress and psychosommatic disorders alienated lots of people in the audience, and we let them know it. Since I didn't have high expectations for the meeting, I was not disappointed.

The most important information for me came from an environmental advocacy group up Broadway from me—they did a Freedom of Information filing with the EPA, New York State, and New York City. Yesterday they got a huge file from the EPA that contains findings which appear to be wildly at variance with what they're putting out publicly. This group hasn't had time to go through the many inches of reports but it seems clear that there's lots of bad things going on down here—again no surprise, as is the fact the State denied them their records because it is a crime scene and NYC asked for 24 more days to respond. As expected, no one in the audience believed the experts—they believed in their noses, they believed in the fires. And they told the experts that they had to do better—which, being clueless academics, they won't be able to.

Almost a month later, on November 1, 2001, the New York City Council held another hearing, which ended in plans for yet another. The same story line seemed to be emerging: while the smoke plume continued to rise, locals were getting sick but the air, according to the experts, was safe. The locals were skeptical of the experts and the experts, while sympathetic, largely dismissive that the dust cloud was causing any serious illness. Policy makers were left in a quandary over what to do.

Community Knowledge and Environmental Health Controversies

Stories like these are not unique. Something unexpected happens, unexplained health problems arise, and residents want some assurance that they are not in danger. While residents share stories, scientists and technicians attempt to show, using techniques such as risk assessment, that no strong causal connections exist between the dangers residents perceive and the health problems that worry them. Policy makers, administrators, and city planners are often left to decide who to believe and what course of action to take.

Should a community defer to professionals, trusting that the findings are accurate and that they are sharing all the information they have? Do professionals have an obligation to take account of community-generated information and to incorporate it, somehow, into their formal analyses? Should local accounts of health risk ever trump expert knowledge? Can we imagine a situation in which we should *not* put our lives and community well-being in the hands of technical experts? Or, would relying on community assessments of environmental health inevitably lead to inadequate protection because locals tend to ignore regional, national, and global factors that influence health?

This book addresses these questions by highlighting the ways in which community-generated information can, in fact, be used to improve environmental health decision-making. Many communities, particularly disadvantaged groups seeking environmental justice, are increasingly rejecting the idea that professional scientists should be left alone to define, analyze, and prescribe solutions for the environmental health hazards they face. Instead, these groups are demanding meaningful participation in assessments and decisions, and pragmatic action to improve community health. *Street Science* follows one such community and reveals how residents organized community knowledge to improve scientific inquiry and environmental health decision making. The book offers a new framework for environmental health justice that joins local insights with professional techniques, a combination that I call "street science." This book shows that "street science" does not devalue science, but rather re-values forms of knowledge that professional science has excluded and democratizes the inquiry and decision-making processes.

The book begins from the position that understanding the links between environmental pollution and public-health problems no longer can be viewed as purely technical problems to be left exclusively to professionals. Concerned lay publics, especially the most disadvantaged populations experiencing the greatest risks and health problems, are demanding a greater role in researching, describing, and prescribing solutions for the hazards they face. When local experience conflicts with the conclusions of experts, residents often question how professionals create, define, and prioritize "problems" and which problems warrant attention. Communities are demanding to "speak for themselves." By drawing on their firsthand experience—here called local knowledge—they are engaging in their own brand of science. This new science puts pressure on environmental and public-health decision makers to find new ways of fusing the expertise of professional practitioners and scientists with the "contextual intelligence" that only local residents possess. This book takes a realistic look at what local knowledge can contribute to the general knowledge base of policymaking and highlights the ways local knowledge differs from professional knowledge. Through detailed examples of community-based environmental-health problem solving I describe how *street science* operates in practice. Generalizing from these cases, the book offers a framework for *street science* that fuses local and professional knowledge with the aim of achieving environmental health justice.

Typically, research into environmental-health decision making asks how science *influences* policy. Science is seen as "speaking truth" to controversial environmental and human-health-risk decision making. In this view, politics is seen as a separate entity that is informed by science. Scientific knowledge is thus presumed to be shaped outside institutional, cultural, and historical contexts—not something integral to and evolving with political decision making. *Street Science* challenges this idea and instead suggests that scientific knowledge is always "co-produced"; science and politics are interdependent, each drawing from the other in a dynamic iterative process. Before further defining the "co-production" of scientific expertise, the book highlights why community knowledge should become an integral part of environmental-health problem solving.

Why Study Local Knowledge?

Street Science engages several issues that remain largely unaddressed in the environmental-policy and public-health literatures. First, increasing evidence suggests that local knowledge has contributed positively to the formulation of more sustainable resource-management practices and development decisions, especially in the developing world (Brush 1980; Chambers 1997; Scott 1998). Yet, little work has examined how this type of knowledge might improve environmental decisions in Western contexts. In developing countries, Andean potato farmers, Indian foresters, and Haitian community-health workers have revealed how their "indigenous knowledge" improved the local environment, development, and human-health conditions. (Van der Ploeg 1993; de Guchteneire et al. 1999; Farmer 1999). Even the World Bank and other international agencies have acknowledged that local people have their own scientific knowledge and practices, and that to assist them professionals must understand something about that knowledge. For example, the 1999 *World Development Report* noted that local knowledge, on par with additional capital, is the key to sustainable social and economic development, reducing poverty, and improving health (World Bank 1999). Surprisingly, little work has explored whether and how local knowledge can be applied in U.S. urban settings where the populations are largely the poor, immigrants, and people of color.

Second, a growing body of literature suggests that inequalities in environmental health, morbidity, and mortality result from a combination of poverty, discrimination, political disenfranchisement, environmental exposures, *and* biologic agents (Evans et al. 1994). The implication of this renewed interest in *social epidemiology* is that disease is less and less believed to be caused by a specific identifiable biological agent and instead that a host of social, economic, political, and biological conditions contribute to well-being (Berkman and Kawachi 2000). Much of this work has recognized that "health" is not just the absence of disease, but the conditions and capabilities—material, physical, social, and biological—that enable populations to make healthy lifestyles choices, avoid disease, and prolong life.[1]

In order to identify these conditions and capabilities, social epidemiologists have turned to the populations suffering the most—such as African-Americans, immigrants, and farm workers—to understand how their daily experiences influence morbidity, mortality, and access to health-promoting resources more generally. The tendency of social epidemiologists has been to turn the "social determinants" of health into covariates in a regression model (Diez-Roux 1998). This quantification of social experience often misses the social contexts, networks and subjective understandings that tell the complex story of what it means to live with environmental exposure and disease burdens (Steingraber 1998). Attention to the meanings people attach to their experiences living in polluted neighborhoods and with persistent disease burdens, and how this experience shapes social action, could further our understanding of inequalities in environmental-health burdens. To extend the work of social epidemiology, this book explores how the local knowledge of disadvantaged populations can influence both the research and decision-making agendas attempting to reverse the health inequalities afflicting residents of urban America.

Third, public health has a rich history of studying how *place*—the geographic areas where we live, learn, work, and play—structures population health. From the work of nineteenth century Europeans such as Edwin Chadwick, Rudolf Virchow, and Fredrick Engels, to the efforts of early American reformers such as Alice Hamilton and Florence Kelley, there was a recognition that the condition of one's neighborhood, housing, and workplace helped explain differences in life expectancy and morbidity among different class, racial, and ethnic groups (Krieger 2001; MacIntyre et al. 1993). The recent revival of "place-focused" public health emphasizes how, for example, neighborhoods and the "built environment" structure health status, not act merely as background to other lifestyle or risk factors (MacIntyre et al. 2002). Place is central to the study of health inequalities because place is increasingly understood as the primary site where the impact of macro-social structures are played out in everyday life (Fitzpatrick and LaGory 2000; Fullilove 2004). *Street Science* shows that local knowledge is a crucial resource for understanding how neighborhoods structure both physical and social exposures, and how street science can assist epidemiologists and policy makers in structuring effective place-based interventions.

Fourth, while environmental-justice activists, some agency staff, and many intergovernmental institutions around the world have "rediscovered" the importance of local knowledge in environmental-health decision making, along with this recognition has come a tendency to romanticize local knowledge as always in harmony with natural and human systems and as superior to other ways of knowing (Agarwal 1995; Warren et al. 1993). Compelling evidence shows that local knowledge can sometimes lead to naive or even detrimental environmental, public health, and development decisions (Buege 1996; Milton 1996). In addition, some commentators suggest that the "rediscovery" of local knowledge is a way to shift the burden of proof to resource-starved residents and exonerate the state's responsibility to protect the least well-off (Gibbs 1994; Krimsky 1984). Others claim that focusing on localism can serve as a smoke screen for political control by private interests. While conflating local knowledge with private interests is without merit, particularly in community-based environmental-health controversies, local knowledge in environmental-health problem-solving is both valuable and limited.

Fifth, one difficulty that local knowledge presents is that its insights are often very contextual, while policymaking tends to make general rules. Much of the work on local knowledge is ethnographic and deeply contextual, and few general patterns or lessons are offered. Advocates of local knowledge have been understandably hesitant to "scale up" or generalize their findings and insights—largely out of fear of inaccurate decontextualizations, oversimplifications, and unjustified generalizations.[2] One result is that professional decision makers have not found ways to incorporate the important understandings from studies of local knowledge into the more generalized practice of policymaking. Scaling up knowledge from local settings to more general policy is a necessary task in environmental health because of the extreme heterogeneity in ecosystems and human-environment linkages. But local knowledge can be used to improve environmental-health decisions while maintaining a heightened sensitivity to the contextually specific qualities of this knowledge.

Finally, the fields of urban planning and public health have increasingly embraced the importance of "local," "public," and bottom-up, as opposed to top-down, approaches to research and decision making (Healey 1997; Minkler 1997; Israel et al. 1998). This view is reflected in practices such as community-based participatory research (CBPR) and community planning (Minkler and Wallerstein 2003; Forester 1999). One aim of these approaches is to enhance the democratic character of decisions by challenging the technocratic model of public decision making. Advocates of these approaches reject the "deficit" model of citizen participation, which assumes that the public is largely ignorant and in need of education regarding environmental and scientific problem solving, and instead embrace a "complementary" model (Wynne 1991). The complementary view assumes that citizens have political rather than technical insight, so citizens are asked to offer values while experts retain autonomy over technical issues. This misses what practitioners and analysts of local knowledge have come to understand, namely that technical expertise is "co-produced" (Jasanoff and Wynne 1998; Susskind and Elliot 1983). I borrow the term *co-production* from the field of science and technology studies and use it here to suggest that scientific knowledge and political order are interdependent and evolve jointly. Yet, how the fusing of different kinds of knowledge occurs in the co-production process rarely has been examined in community-based environmental-health controversies.

Situating Street Science

While street science is a practice of knowledge production that embraces the co-production framework (and a process further defined in chapter 2 and throughout the book), it is worth mentioning from the outset that street science is also a process that builds on a number of existing participatory models of knowing and doing. *Street science* ought to be conceptualized as a process that encompasses many of the key principles of the broad set of participatory research methods increasingly called participatory-action research and community-based participatory research. However, street science differs from these techniques by not taking as a priori truths the meanings and definitions of issues framed by professionals. Many participatory-research processes aim to make the *methods* of inquiry more legitimate by opening up participation to lay persons and giving community members an opportunity to prioritize issues. They also tend to create processes for building public consensus around research results and interpretations, and involve these same publics in action to improve their situation. Rarely are problem definitions, meanings, and purposes open for negotiation or reframing by lay people in these processes. Street science, by embracing the co-production model of expertise, is a process that emphasizes the need to open up both problem framing and subsequent methods of inquiry to local knowledge and community participation. Street science raises the contentious political questions that professional "techno-science" tries to silence by often claiming that an issue is "purely technical." Importantly, street science should be thought of as an overarching process that embraces many of the ideals from action research, community-based participatory research, popular epidemiology, and joint fact-finding, but differs from each of these in significant ways.

The driving concept in action research is that information gathering and knowledge production ought to start by engaging in and changing practice (Dewey 1944; Horton 1998; Brown and Tandon 1983). The idea might be described as turning the traditional research paradigm of "ready-aim-fire" (i.e., hypothesis, tests, new theory) on its head; "fire-aim-ready" (action, methods, theory). Street science embraces the action-research idea of starting with practice, but rejects this model for failing to explicitly challenge the deficit model.

Participatory action research (PAR) attempts to make action research more democratic by emphasizing that the individuals and groups impacted by an action must be involved in practice (Chambers 1997; Freire 1974; Whyte 1943, 1991; Fals Borda and Rahman 1991). PAR also recognizes that actions often are more effectively implemented and more likely to meet the needs of a population if these same people are involved in problem solving. This process does not specify how to manage potential conflicts between professional knowledge and that of other participants, particularly lay people. While the "practitioners" in PAR are often professionals and lay people—often the poor and people of color—how to engage a specific group of lay people is generally not specified. This model differs from street science because it tends to embrace the complementary, not the co-production, model.

Community-based participatory research (CBPR) embraces the action paradigm of PAR and specifies that community members, particularly from underserved groups and/or geographic areas, are crucial participants and that action ought to be oriented toward community improvement (Israel et al. 1998; Minkler and Wallerstein 2003). In addition, CBPR emphasizes "capacity building" of community members (i.e., participants are better off after the process), improving relationships between community members and "outsiders" (i.e., government agencies, academics, other professionals), and incorporating local knowledge into the research process. CBPR models tend to adhere to the overarching objectives of the sponsoring organization (such as academics operating under a research grant) and structure community participation to address these predetermined objectives.

These definitions reflect the prevailing tendencies for each practice, and little agreement exists even among practitioners of these methods. For example, the National Institute of Environmental Health Sciences (NIEHS) and the Kellogg Foundation have both emphasized the importance of CBPR for reshaping environmental-health research and addressing health disparities (Kellogg Foundation 2003; O'Fallon and Dearry 2002; O'Fallon et al. 2003). While the NIEHS definition of CBPR emphasizes "information sharing," Kellogg's stresses the creation of "learning communities." For some practitioners, the NIEHS CBPR framework might imply one-way information exchange while Kellogg's paradigm demands dynamic two-way communication that includes long-term relationship building.

Popular epidemiology is another form of CBPR that closely resembles street science (Brown and Mikkelsen 1990). Brown defines *popular epidemiology* as the process where lay people "gather scientific data and other information and also direct and marshal the knowledge and resources of experts in order to understand the epidemiology of disease" (1992, 269). While street science embraces many of the ideas and methods of popular epidemiology, it is a process that is not limited to epidemiological investigations or methods. As this book shows, street scientists can question the appropriate research and action frameworks for the questions they decide are important to study. Street science also encompasses a wider spectrum of questions and methods than popular epidemiology. For example, the case studies in this book show that street scientists often question whether "epidemiology" and "risk" are the right frames around which to structure research and intervention strategies. Street science also embraces a wider range of legitimate knowledge-making and communication techniques than popular epidemiology. For example, street scientists might use street murals, hand-drawn maps, and other images to understand and communicate what they know.

Finally, street science builds from a collaborative method of resolving public scientific disputes called *joint fact-finding* (Ehrmann and Stinson 1999; Ozawa 1991). Most often used when technical issues are in dispute, joint fact-finding is a process that makes explicit that science-intensive controversies involve value judgments, that a range of stakeholder interests must be involved in data gathering and analysis, and that environmental dispute-resolution techniques, including neutral mediation, should be used to assist stakeholders in resolving controversies. Professional analysts from a range of disciplines usually are selected by the mediator and other stakeholders to represent interests from the private sector, government, academia, and nongovernmental organizations (NGOs). While joint fact-finding does not have an explicit community-action orientation, nor does it necessarily include participants from disadvantaged communities, the collaborative method provides a framework for how professional and lay knowledge might be fused in environmental-health problem solving. However, for joint fact-fining to embody the ideals of street science, the process must explicitly embrace the social-justice components of some of the other collaborative methods mentioned above.

This book speaks to researchers, policy makers, and planners and calls on them to stop being so bureaucratic and instead become "reflective practitioners" (Schon 1983). Professionals must learn how to view their practice in a more open-ended way, managing uncertainty by acknowledging the limits to their expertise and meaningfully valuing other kinds of knowledge. Such open-ended engagement requires a special kind of interaction with community members, especially those bearing the brunt of society's ills. As public administrators, especially urban planners, are increasingly forced to play a mediating role between scientists, policy makers, and various publics, they will need to learn new ways of taking account of the local knowledge embedded in the communities within which they work. *Street Science* offers a way for environmental-health decisions to draw from the best science has to offer while also upholding the democratic ideals of participation and justice.

Science on the Streets of Brooklyn

In the most unlikely of communities—a low-income community of color in the Greenpoint/Williamsburg neighborhood of Brooklyn, New York—residents are *doing science*. Using their experiences from living with years of toxic exposures and poor health, residents in this community have organized their knowledge to supplement what professional researchers and decision makers have to say about their neighborhood. The accounts, stories, tests, and practices of residents represent what I am calling *local knowledge*. Generally, *local knowledge* can be understood as the scripts, images, narratives, and understandings we use to make sense of the world in which we live. When combined with insights, tools, and techniques from disciplinary science, local knowledge forms the basis of *street science*. While this book focuses on street science performed by residents of this one Brooklyn neighborhood, the findings are relevant for communities everywhere seeking to understand the environmental-health hazards they face and for professional researchers and decision makers seeking to improve the democratic character of science-based policymaking.

The Greenpoint/Williamsburg Neighborhood, Brooklyn, New York

The Greenpoint/Williamsburg (G/W) section of Brooklyn, New York (figure I.1), is one of the most polluted communities in New York City (NYC). Defined by Brooklyn Community Board 1, G/W has approximately 160,000 residents living in an area of less than five square miles. These residents are some of the poorest in all of New York City, with 35.7 percent of the G/W population living below the poverty line (U.S. Bureau of Census 2000). The median household income for the neighborhood is $16,409, compared to $25,684 for Brooklyn as a whole, and $29,805 for New York City generally. In addition to poverty, only 43.7 percent of adults over twenty-four years old have a high school diploma or higher level of education, compared with averages of 63.7 percent in Brooklyn and 68.3 percent in New York City generally. The ethnically diverse neighborhood is approximately 42 percent Latino (mostly Puerto Rican and Dominican), 24 percent Hasidic Jew, 13 percent African-American, and 10 percent Polish and Slavic immigrant (figure I.2).

The G/W neighborhood also has the largest proportion of land (12 percent) devoted to industrial uses of any of New York City's fifty-nine community districts (Perris and Chait 1998). The average percentage of industrial land use for all districts in the City is 1.9 percent (Perris and

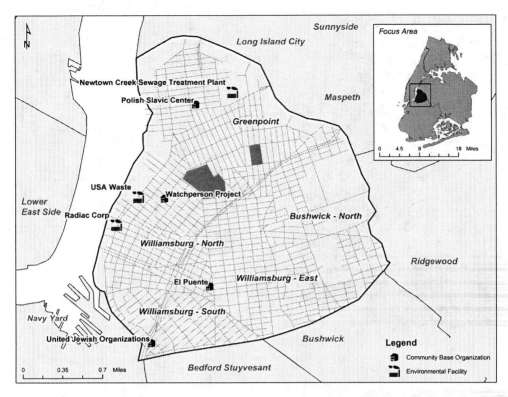

Figure I.1.
Greenpoint/Williamsburg neighborhood, Brooklyn, New York. Source: CMAP/
OASIS, http://www.oasisnyc.net/mapsearch.asp.

Chait 1998). The neighborhood houses a disproportionate number of
polluting facilities, including: the Newtown Creek sewage treatment
plant; thirty solid-waste transfer stations, where garbage is stored before
transported to landfill; a radioactive waste storage facility; over thirty
facilities which store extremely hazardous wastes, seventeen petroleum
and natural-gas storage facilities; and ninety-six aboveground oil-storage
tanks (figure I.3) (NYC DEP 1997). In 1987 a study by Hunter College's
Community Environmental Health Center, called *Right-to-Breathe,
Right-to-Know,* revealed that Williamsburg was home to the largest concentration of Toxic Release Inventory–reporting industries in New York
City (Steinsapir et al. 1992). Not much had changed ten years later. In
1997 the community housed sixty facilities storing, using, or manufac-

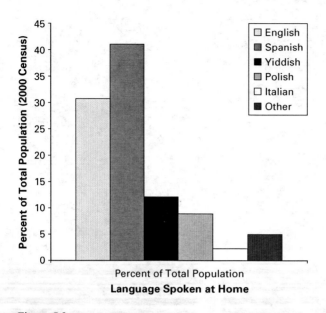

Figure I.2.
Primary language spoken at home, Greenpoint/Williamsburg neighborhood, Brooklyn, New York. Source: 2000 U.S. Census File SF3a.

turing 10,000 pounds or more of a hazardous substance, 161 facilities reporting hazardous substances in the Citywide Facility Inventory Database, 21 Toxic Release Inventory (TRI) facilities, and 11 facilities using or storing extremely hazardous materials with Risk Management Plans (NYC DEP 1997). With these numbers, G/W ranks first out of all community districts in New York City for housing the highest number of these facilities (NYC DEP 1997).

One result of the concentration of polluting facilities in the neighborhood is elevated levels of localized hazardous air pollutants (HAPs). A 1999 EPA study modeling 148 HAPs in the neighborhood at the census-tract level found that concentrations of 17 HAPs exceeded EPA health-benchmark levels (table I.1), which are equivalent to a one-in-a-million lifetime cancer risk. These same air toxics were found to be greater than those estimated in 75 percent and sometimes 95 percent of all U.S. census tracts and all NYC area census tracts (US EPA 1999a).

Using the HAP exposures outlined in table I.1, the EPA compared the toxicity-weighted cumulative HAP exposure for G/W to cumulative

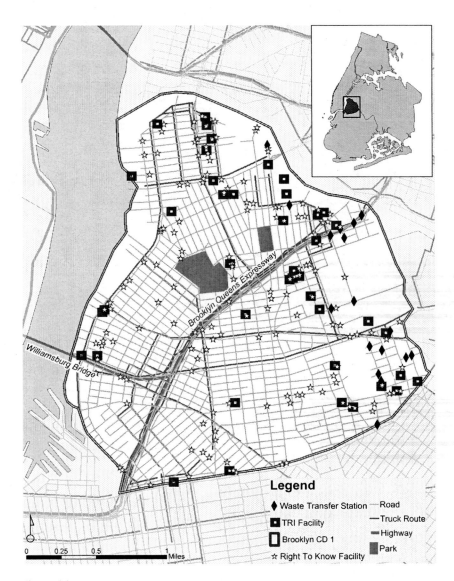

Figure I.3.
Environmental hazards in Greenpoint/Williamsburg neighborhood. Source:
PICCED and G/W 197a Plan, http://www.gwapp.org/197.html.

Table I.1
Hazardous Air Pollutants Exceeding Health-Benchmark Levels

Chemical Name	Average concentration (µg/m³)	EPA health-benchmark level (µg/m³)	Ranking of G/W HAP concentrations compared to those found in all U.S. census tracts	Ranking of G/W HAP concentrations compared to those found in all NYC-area census tracts
Acetaldehyde	3.0	0.45	Top 5%	Top 25%
Acrolein	1.0	0.02	Top 5%	Top 25%
Acrylonitrile	**0.002**	**0.015**	**Top 5%**	**Top 5%**
Arsenic	0.001	0.00023	Top 25%	
Benzene	**6.0**	**0.12**	**Top 5%**	**Top 25%**
1,3-butadiene	0.6	0.0036	Top 5%	Top 25%
Carbon tetrachloride	0.9	0.067	Top 25%	Top 25%
Chloroform	0.1	0.043	Top 25%	Top 25%
Chromium (VI)	**0.0004**	**0.000083**	**Top 25%**	**Top 5%**
p-dichlorobenzene	0.5	0.091	Top 5%	Top 25%
1,3-dichloropropene	0.2	0.063	Top 5%	
Ethylene dichloride	**0.2**	**0.038**	**Top 25%**	**Top 5%**
Formaldehyde	5.0	0.077	Top 5%	Top 25%
Methyl chloride	1.0	0.56		Top 25%
Nickel	0.04	0.005	Top 5%	
PCDD/PCDFs	0.0000001	0.00000003	Top 5%	Top 25%
Vinyl Chloride	**0.1**	**0.012**	**Top 5%**	**Top 5%**

Source: US EPA 1999a.

HAP exposures for the nation as a whole, urban areas throughout the nation, and the greater NYC area (US EPA 1999a, ch. 6, p. 11). The EPA analyses revealed that the cumulative HAP exposure in G/W is over 360 times greater than that which would result in a one-in-a-million risk of cancer, over 3 times higher than estimated national exposures, nearly 2.5 times greater than exposures in U.S. urban areas, and 1.3 times higher than exposure in the greater NYC area.

Residents also are exposed to heavy vehicular traffic and mobile-source pollution from the Brooklyn-Queens Expressway (BQE), an elevated roadway that bisects the community. Mobil Oil Corporation has recovered over 5.19 million gallons of petroleum product from underneath 52 acres of the neighborhood. This product resulted from years of negligent operations at neighborhood storage-tank farms. Finally, only 3.0 percent of the neighborhood is shaded by trees, compared to an average of 11.4 percent tree cover for all Brooklyn neighborhoods and an average coverage of 16.6 percent for all NYC neighborhoods (Perris and Chait 1998).

Despite the plethora of hazards in the neighborhood, few public health studies have focused on G/W. A report by the NYC Public Advocate's office in 1998 entitled *Lead and Kids* indicated that between 1994 and 1998, G/W ranked in the top 12 (out of 30) NYC health districts in number of new cases of children with blood lead levels at or above 10 micrograms per deciliter (10 µg/dl), set by the Centers for Disease Control (CDC) the maximum safe standard (Green 1998). The New York City Department of Environmental Protection (NYCDEP) supported two neighborhood-health studies of G/W focusing on rates of cancer, asthma, birth defects, and childhood lead poisoning; they found the elevated rates of cancer in the community statistically significant to cause alarm (table I.2) (Kaminsky et al. 1992). These studies did not find any significantly elevated prevalence of asthma or birth defects. However, the asthma study was limited to hospitalization rates and the birth-defects study reviewed data from only one local hospital, suggesting that these results may not capture the entire picture (Kaminsky et al. 1992).

The environmental justice (EJ) movement has highlighted how low-income communities and communities of color, often in urban areas, face disproportionate hazardous exposures and elevated rates of morbid-

Table I.2
Statistically Significant Cancers in the Greenpoint/Williamsburg Neighborhood and their Ranking for all N.Y.C. Health Districts

Cancer type	Rank—based on incidence between 1978–1987, all Community District 1 census tracks, and compared to all NYC Health districts (30 total Districts)			
	Male children under 15 yrs	Female children under 15 yrs	Women over 15 yrs	Men over 15 yrs
All cancers	2nd	N/A	N/A	N/A
Total leukemias	1st	7th	N/A	N/A
Leukemia (unspecified)	3rd	1st	N/A	N/A
Acute lymphocytic leukemia (ALL)	2nd	N/A	N/A	N/A
Acute myelogenous leukemia (AML)	2nd	N/A	N/A	2nd
Chronic myelogenous leukemia (CML)	4th	N/A	N/A	3rd
Nervous system	3rd	N/A	N/A	2nd
Stomach	N/A	N/A	1st	1st
Lung	N/A	N/A	N/A	8th
Pancreas	N/A	N/A	3rd	N/A

Source: Kaminsky et al. 1992.

ity and mortality (Bullard 1994; Cole and Foster 2000). Many residents in these communities, similar to G/W, lack a formal education, and the neighborhoods tend to have different cultural subcommunities, most of which have distinct languages, practices, and lifestyles. These same urban communities, also like G/W, simultaneously bear the hazardous exposures typical of a declining industrial and manufacturing base, and the economic and housing instability that often accompanies this decline. Thus, an analysis of how residents of the G/W neighborhood grapple with environmental health burdens, can be generalized to an examination of how street science can help pursue environmental-health justice in disadvantaged urban communities everywhere.

The Case Studies: Environmental Health Controversies in Brooklyn

This book follows four separate episodes in Brooklyn's Greenpoint/ Williamsburg neighborhood in which community members organized around an environmental health hazard, engaged with the science of environmental health, and challenged either the diagnosis or prescription offered by professionals. The four episodes were selected because they each deal with some of the most pressing environmental health issues facing low-income communities in the United States, such as asthma and childhood lead poisoning. The range of issues covered in each case also highlights that community members are capable of learning about and engaging in a number of complex scientific and policy problems. The four cases also highlight that street science is not one practice but a set of diverse practices, that community scientists partner with professionals differently, and that street science evolves in a community over many years of struggle. Finally, the cases reveal both the successes and limitations of street science and each takes a realistic look at the contributions of community knowledge to environmental-health justice.

Exploring how these community members engage in the practice of street science shows how lay people often seek to supplement and ultimately transform professional views about what is happening in their community. The street scientists working on the streets of Brooklyn do not seek to dismiss professional science outright, but rather explore how to change that science from the inside by partnering with professionals and revealing that community members are credible experts in their own right. The four episodes include risks from subsistence fish diets, high rates of asthma, childhood lead poisoning, and risks from local air-pollution sources.

Subsistence Fishing Risks

Reacting to pressure from the environmental-justice movement, the EPA decided to pilot its cumulative-exposure project in the G/W community. The EPA held a series of meetings to inform the community about the assessment. At one meeting, residents and community organizations reacted in shock after the EPA informed them that the dietary portion of the assessment would use a "default urban diet." Residents told the agency that the Latino, Caribbean African-American, Polish immigrant, and Hasidic Jewish residents that lived in the neighborhood did not have the typical "urban diet." In addition, residents informed the agency that many community members were eating fish from the East River. The EPA had no data on this potentially toxic exposure, and since many of the anglers were poor, non-English speakers and Caribbean immigrants, they would be reluctant to speak with outsiders. One community group, The Watchperson Project, convinced the EPA that they should gather information on angler practices so that this exposure could be included in the assessment. The EPA and the Watchperson Project worked together to develop a survey and interview protocol, and the community organization organized volunteers to interview the anglers. The survey gathered information on the type and amount of fish residents were eating, the age of fish consumers, and their ethnicity. This information was presented to the EPA and incorporated into its exposure assessment. The project eventually led to fishing advisories, multilingual educational campaigns, and the construction of a community garden to provide an alternative for inexpensive food. The episode reveals how local knowledge can improve assessments of the multiple and cumulative burdens that typically afflict residents of urban neighborhoods. The case also exemplifies how community residents can gather important information about potential neighborhood hazards that regulatory agencies and scientists often overlook, that information is often embedded in cultural practices, and that street science often supplements, but does not replace, professional analyses.

Asthma Epidemic in the Latino Community
A high school science-class project monitoring air pollution and neighborhood health sparked interest at El Puente, a community organization, to address alarming rates of asthma in the neighborhood. The student project led to a community-health survey and to a partnership between El Puente and the nonprofit organization Community Information and Epidemiological Technologies (CIET). Since 1995, El Puente and CIET have undertaken a series of health surveys focusing on local asthma rates, possible causes, and health-management practices of the neighborhood's Latino population. The project has employed residents, mostly non-English speaking Latinas, as community health workers (CHWs). The

CHWs have helped design and perform the health surveys, lead focus-group meetings to interpret the survey findings, and provided basic health-maintenance information through door-to-door outreach to suffering residents. El Puente's surveys, focus groups, and community organizing have tapped local knowledge previously unknown to outside health-care providers, pointing out surprising findings such as the prevalence of asthma among older women, how locals view professional asthma treatments, and the use of cultural and religious-based home remedies for treating asthma. This knowledge contributed to local interventions, such as enrolling residents in free health insurance, educating physicians on the cultural medicinal practices of local Latinos, and developing asthma-management plans for those with the disease. The episode details how local knowledge improves community-based research partnerships between neighborhood organizations and public health professionals.

Childhood Lead Poisoning
When city workers began sandblasting lead-based paint off the Williamsburg Bridge with no screens to capture the paint, community members reacted by organizing residents to determine whether the paint chips were a health hazard. After measuring lead dust and neighborhood children's blood for lead and finding some elevated levels, residents sued the city to stop the sandblasting. Subsequent soil tests around the bridge found highly contaminated soil. Residents organized the Williamsburg Around the Bridge Block Association (WABBA) and the city, reacting to pressure from the community, media, and elected officials, convened a task force to address the elevated blood and soil levels and to devise new guidelines for bridge sandblasting. After three years of negotiations and lawsuits, the State Supreme Court ruled that the city had to perform an environmental and public-health review of the bridge sandblasting. As part of the settlement, the city was instructed to fund a team of health experts, chosen by WABBA, to assist the community in participating in the review process. This episode reviews the face-to-face interactions between the professional consultants and the community, the challenges community residents encounter describing their local knowledge to professionals who might be sympathetic to their concerns but who also question local people's methods, and the difficulties of doing street

science when decision-making forums and models are limited to those defined by professionals.

Air Pollution and Mapping Local Knowledge

The proposed siting of a solid waste incinerator in the neighborhood galvanized a group of high school students to form a group called the Toxic Avengers. The students helped organize residents to attend a public hearing and brought Latinos and Jews in the neighborhood together for the first time. An environmental town meeting was held to educate and organize residents to oppose the incinerator. The Toxic Avengers made a map entitled "Our Town" depicting the numerous environmental health hazards in the community. Out of the town meeting came the Community Alliance For the Environment (CAFE), the first multiethnic environmental coalition in the neighborhood and a key force in defeating the incinerator. The community eventually developed its own geographic information system (GIS) and generated its own maps. In one instance, the Watchperson Project used their maps to challenge the city's approval of the largest waste-transfer station on the East Coast. The community's map supported its argument at a public hearing, at which it challenged the anticipated cumulative environmental impacts in the neighborhood. In another case, the community-generated GIS maps revealed to the EPA that its dispersion model for hazardous air pollutants neglected to include thousands of small-source polluters in the neighborhood. The EPA model was intended to model exposures to hazardous air pollutants at the census-tract level, but the community's maps showed how the concentration of air polluters changed from block-to-block and even along the same city block. This episode highlights the importance of and limitations to using visual tools, particularly maps, for performing street science.

Research Methods

These cases presented reflect a range of research methods used over the course of six years, from 1996 to 2002, in order to understand the street science of Brooklyn residents. From 1996 to 1998, I was a senior environmental planner with the NYC DEP, and I spent much of my professional time investigating hazards in the G/W community and working with professionals and residents to understand and address the community's environmental-health concerns. During this time I was a participant-observer in public meetings and focus groups that were held during each of the four episodes. I also attended other public meetings where local residents were key participants and environmental-health information gathered by locals was discussed. These public meetings included the Newtown Creek Citizens Advisory Council, Brooklyn Community Board 1 meetings, and NYCDEP's Environmental Benefits Program meetings. While at the NYCDEP, I participated in a number of environmental-health analyses of the G/W community, including the environmental-impact assessment for the Newtown Creek sewage-treatment plant, the Williamsburg Bridge repainting, and the analysis of the USA Waste transfer station.

As a doctoral student at MIT from 1998 to 2002, I returned to the neighborhood as a researcher. During this time, I conducted numerous one-on-one structured interviews, both in person and via telephone, with community members and professionals working in the community. I also "shadowed" activists and community researchers for weeks at a time, observing how they engaged in inquiry. My methodology included "street ethnography," or unstructured interviews and conversations with community residents about the issues and processes discussed in the book. During this same time I reviewed primary texts, such as internal memos, and documents from community-based organizations, private consultants, and the government agencies involved in each of the four cases. The government documents included environmental-impact statements, court documents, and other planning studies performed in the neighborhood by the NYC Mayor's Office of Environmental Coordination, the NYC Departments of Environmental Protection, City Planning, Sanitation, and Law, the New York State Department of Environmental Conservation, and the U.S. Environmental Protection Agency. Finally, I also reviewed newspaper and other popular-press articles on the neighborhood.

Chapter Overviews

Chapter 1, Local Knowledge in Environmental Health Policy, introduces a key tension that can arise in environmental health problem solving when professionals aim to use the latest scientific expertise and models while they are simultaneously committed to democratic, participatory decision making. The chapter reviews, engages, and critiques the key conceptual debates over this tension in the policy sciences, public health, and risk literatures. It highlights how decision makers miss information that can improve scientific outcomes and the fairness of decision making when they fail to account for what populations living with a hazard already know.

Chapter 2, Street Science: The Characteristics of Local Knowledge, provides a detailed introduction to and definition of what I mean by *local knowledge* and how it acts as the foundation of a form of scientific inquiry that I call *street science*. The chapter includes three vignettes from environmental-health conflicts around the world describing how lay people have used their knowledge to improve environmental-health problem solving. The chapter provides examples of street science, reveals how local knowledge differs from that of professionals, and highlights the general characteristics of local knowledge that make it a useful category for environmental-health decision making.

Chapters 3–6 present four "street science episodes" from the Greenpoint/Williamsburg neighborhood. They all describe the benefits and limits of the street-science process in different environmental-health decision-making contexts.

The last chapter, Street Science: Toward Environmental Health Justice, draws the key policymaking lessons for street science, pulling from the four episodes. It suggests how street science confronts inequitable distributions of power in the science-policymaking process and some conditions that make the street science of community members successful with professionals. It includes a discussion of the epistemological contribution local knowledge makes to environmental-health decision making. The book concludes with recommendations for community members seeking environmental-health justice and for professional practitioners committed to technically sound and democratically robust problem solving.

1

Local Knowledge in Environmental Health Policy

The Tensions between Communities and Professionals

How do environmental-health professionals typically deal with a situation like the controversy over air quality and public health after the World Trade Center collapse described in the introduction? Typically, environmental health seeks to identify the specific pollutants in the medium of concern. In this example, scientists attempt to delineate the individual toxins in the air. Once the pollutants are identified, they are assessed for their toxicity, or their potential danger and deleterious effects on humans generally. Next, each individual pollutant identified is assessed for its potential impact on humans exposed to the air pollution from the World Trade Center. Determinations of human-health impacts in a specific place generally include assumptions about the routes of exposure (e.g., inhalation in the case of air pollution), how much pollution certain groups are inhaling (e.g., children versus construction workers), and how long certain groups are exposed. The toxicity information and the exposure assumptions are combined to estimate the human-health risk from each individual pollutant contained in the World Trade Center air. This process of identifying each hazard and its toxicity to humans, estimating an individual's exposure to the hazard in a particular place, and extrapolating from this information an estimate of potential harm, is called *risk assessment*.

Risk has been the dominant frame through which environmental health is analyzed in the United States for at least the last thirty years (Fiorino 1989).[3] Risk, and its correlate risk assessment, implies that a problem can be clearly defined, quantified, and therefore managed. Once some version of health risk is generated, the "benefits" from the source of the pollution or hazard are weighed against the pollution's "costs" to human health. At this stage, policy analysts and planners are charged with the often inevitable task of "risk management," or deciding how to weigh "costs and benefits" and inform policymaking.[4]

In the best risk-management processes, the analyst consults with the public that is being asked to bear a "risk" from the beginning of the hazard assessment (Krimsky and Plough 1988). However, more often analysts—perhaps feeling that professional training gives them ultimate discretion to carry out and implement decisions—omit the public from the decision-making process. Additionally, the analysts may find it difficult to divine what the scientists really found in their study, how the legislature, governor, or mayor wants the "costs and benefits" to be interpreted and administered, and what course is consistent with the "public interest." The analysts may feel that their agency is "captured" by private interest groups that are seeking to influence the analysis and any resulting regulation (Lowi 1969). The "captured agency" then might substitute private goals for those of the public at large because the constituency opposing the private sector may not be organized, the agency may rely on the private sector for resources necessary to implement particular programs, or because of the powerful influence industry has in local, state, and national politics.

In the midst of these potentially conflicting interests, the analysts or planners often decide that the tacit operating rule is that the best public is a quiescent one. The analysts might desire to faithfully represent the values and interests of citizens but be unsure what "representation" actually entails. They may ask whether political representation requires that an agency allow local people to participate in analyses and decision making. Recognizing that the success of environmental-health policy is often contingent on the willingness of ordinary citizens to accept the validity of official policy framings, the analysts might hold a public hearing. Hearings tend to open up to unlimited critical scrutiny expert findings that were generated in closed worlds of formal inquiry. These processes are often recipes for unending debate and spiraling distrust, leaving most participants unsatisfied and frustrated that, for instance, technical uncertainties were left unresolved. Thus, the planners may be torn between holding a public hearing that might merely act as a forum to placate the demands of competing special interests groups or organizing some other public process that they have no experience in managing. Public officials, unsure of how to deal with these tensions and competing commitments, often try to work quietly, get the job done without disturbing the public "peace," and then often reassure everyone "out there" that there is no reason to be concerned or involved (Reich 1988, 124).

This description might oversimplify the risk-management process, but it highlights some of the tensions environmental-health professionals face when determining how best to use scientific analyses while simultaneously committing to democratic decision making.[5] One way to resolve this tension is to return to and challenge the "risk framework" that tends to dominate environmental health. In the risk frame, certain types of evidence and expertise are valued and other evidence and expertise is ignored. The risk frame tends to prefer formal and quantitative information and the participation of a select group of professionals trained in certain disciplines. For example, Jasanoff (1990) has noted how expert advisors in policymaking are chosen based on their technical competence, ability to construct "objective science," and political independence and neutrality. Experts protect their authority to deal with the uncertain science of risk though a sociological mechanism known as "boundary work."

Boundary work is a process where experts assign the array of issues and controversies lying between the two ideal typical poles of "pure science" and "pure policy" to one or the other side of the policy-science boundary (Gieryn 1995, 405). As Jasanoff observes:

When an area of intellectual activity is tagged with the label "science," people who are not scientists are *de facto* barred from having any say about its substance; correspondingly, to label something "not science" [e.g., mere politics] is to denude it of cognitive authority. (Jasanoff 1990, 14)

As a result, risk-based problem framing and decision-making processes largely ignore evidence that is more informal, experiential, tacit, and explicitly value laden (Wynne 1996; Irwin 1995). Lay publics, even when granted "entry" into policymaking through formalized public hearings, are required to offer evidence in a "voice" or language that mirrors that of experts. As a result, the quantitative risk frame in environmental health puts lay publics at a disadvantage from the outset and limits their ability to participate in and influence decisions when compared to scientists and other professionals.

Antecedents to Street Science

Attempts to bring local or lay knowledge into environmental health decision making are not new. From nineteenth-century Progressive Era reformers to 1960s and 1970s anti-toxics activism, today's street scientists are building on ideas and community-based practices that emerged over a century ago (Gottlieb 1993). While taking slightly different approaches and being labeled everything from "shoe-leather epidemiology" to "people's science," community-based science has played a role in shaping environmental-health research and political action. Yet, even before Progressive Era reformers enrolled local knowledge to address the health problems afflicting the urban poor, public-health work in Europe highlighted the importance of considering the social and community aspects of health.

A series of studies in the mid-nineteenth century gave rise to modern movements for community-based environmental health. For example, one of the first modern epidemiological studies of neighborhood health was performed by Louis René Villermé, who used statistics to study Paris neighborhoods in 1840 and demonstrated a clear connection between ill health and neighborhood poverty. In 1848, Rudolf Virchow documented the social causes of a typhus epidemic in Germany. He is credited for linking the biologic, social, and economic underpinnings of health and emphasizing that medicine and public health fail when they ignore the plight of the poor and working class (Rosen 1993).

Perhaps most influential on American reformers was the 1842 publication of Edwin Chadwick's *Report on the Sanitary Conditions of the Laboring Population in Great Britain,* and similar reports that soon followed documenting conditions in New York and Massachusetts (Duffy 1990). These reports stimulated the Sanitary movement in public health and highlighted how inferior living and working environments for the poor and immigrant populations were a key factor in their poor health (Melosi 2000). The Sanitary movement was part of a host of Progressive Era reforms that focused public-health interventions on cleaning up urban neighborhoods and workplaces (Duffy 1990). One of the most well-known reform movements of this time was the Settlement House movement, best exemplified by Hull House in Chicago, where reformers such as Jane Addams, Alice Hamilton, and Florence Kelley founded the modern epidemiologic methods of occupational and community health.

At the time Jane Addams founded Hull House in 1889, pollution in cities and the workplace was seen as a sign of progress and opportunity, not potential harm. In this context, the public-health work by the women at Hull House was revolutionary because it not only challenged this idea, but also because these reformers used research methods that included the lived experiences and knowledge of those experiencing the greatest suffering. The methods of reformers at Hull House applied the information gleaned from workers and community residents to more detailed investigations (Deegan 1990). An important aspect of their public-health philosophy was encouraging community residents to record and share their experiences with others in the community, the general public, and decision makers. As Jane Addams stated in her introduction to the classic 1895 work *Hull House Maps and Papers*:

The residents of Hull-House offer these maps and papers to the public, not as exhaustive treatises, but as recorded observations which may plausibly be of value, because they are immediate, and the result of long acquaintance. (*Hull House Maps and Papers* 1895, vii)

For Addams and others at Hull House, the knowledge community residents provided was a vital resource for both understanding and changing the unhealthy conditions of the urban environment.

Alice Hamilton, one of the first American specialists in the field of occupational disease and a long-term Hull House resident, pioneered the use of local knowledge to inform her work toward ameliorating common workplace hazards of the day, such as mercury poisoning of felt-hat workers and lead poisoning (Hamilton 1943). Refusing to see workers as appropriate guinea pigs for the discovery of the health effects of industrial chemicals, Hamilton listened to workers' accounts of the workplace experience to help her hypothesize why certain occupations and industrial processes were hazardous (Hamilton 1943). While workers often were reluctant to talk out of fear of losing their jobs, Hamilton met them on their own time, visiting homes to conduct informal interviews and to listen to their stories of workplace horrors (Sicherman 1984). Hamilton's style of fieldwork, which came to be known as "shoe-leather epidemiology," helped her piece together dangers in the workplace that were routinely underreported by factory owners and physicians (Sicherman 1984).

Florence Kelley, another Hull House resident, also pioneered the use of local knowledge in environmental health investigations. Kelley, like Hamilton, took her investigations into the street and canvassed the neighborhood around Hull House to document hazardous living conditions. One of her major achievements was documenting the "sweating system," or the dangerous garment-work women and children who lived in tenement houses performed (*Hull House Maps and Papers* 1895, 31).

The work of Addams, Hamilton, Kelley, and other reformers at Hull House aimed to understand how, in an unjust world, health is driven by social and economic inequalities. They understood that in order to change inequitable social conditions, one must first learn from the vulnerable groups how they described their suffering, because these stories hold clues about causes and effective interventions. These pioneers of local knowledge also encouraged the use of lay practitioners, such as midwifes and sanitation inspectors, to supplement the work of physicians and engineers (Deegan 1990). Importantly, women were at the forefront of early community-based social reforms and, as chapters 3–6 show, continue to lead most street science investigations.

While the Progressive Era reforms continued through the early years of the twentieth century, the public support for this work waned as germ theory came to dominate public health. Germ theory held that specific agents of infectious disease exist, in particular microbes, and that these agents correspond one-to-one with specific diseases (Tesh 1988). Research and interventions driven by laboratory investigations of microbes quickly replaced the sanitary, social, and political reforms advocated by Progressive Era reformers. Public-health interventions focused on specific immunization plans, with physicians emerging as the new class of public-health professionals, leaving community organizers and lay people with little room to participate in this expert-centered discourse.

One important exception to this dynamic, where local knowledge was integrated into community health, was the neighborhood-health-center movement that emerged around 1910 but declined rapidly after World

War I. Seeking in part to replicate the success of settlement workers, city governments began "demonstration projects" where health- and welfare-agency work was bought together and relocated "from city hall to the neighborhood" to better serve the neediest populations (Rosen 1985). The neighborhood health center aimed to replicate the values of "acquaintance" with "active participation" of the local population in delivering services that had proved so successful for the Settlement House movement (Bamberger 1966). Health centers were started in immigrant neighborhoods of Milwaukee and Philadelphia, the Mohawk-Brighton district of Cincinnati, New York's Lower East Side, and the West End of Boston. A key component of all the health centers was the creation of block committees, which allowed residents to raise neighborhood-specific problems to the nurses, physicians, and other professionals staffing the center (Burnham 1920). According to Rosen (1985), in a radical step for the time, the health officer for the Lower East Side center was a Jewish physician who understood the people, their language, and culture.

The cessation of large-scale immigration during the war years, and accusations that the self-governing aspects of the health centers were a "Red plot" and "socialized medicine," eliminated municipal support for neighborhood-based health programs (Rosen 1985). In addition, antagonism toward lay involvement in delivering health services by the American Medical Association helped eliminate funding for community-based prenatal and child health services provided for under the Sheppard-Towner Act of 1921 (Meckel 1990). By the 1930s lay participation in community-health issues was almost nonexistent because most epidemiologic investigations ignored social factors or treated them as nuisance variables in statistical models that focused on isolating germs. In the classic epidemiology framework of host-agent-environment, interventions focused on immunizing the "host" (e.g., individuals) because the "environment" (e.g., the world outside of microorganisms) was seen as harder to control.

While professionals increasingly adopted the biomedical model of disease—which attributed morbidity and mortality to individual behaviors, biology, and genetics—impoverished communities organized to address health issues with the help of organizations such as The Highlander Folk School, later renamed the Highlander Research and Education Center, in

Tennessee founded by Myles Horton (Horton 1971). Horton and the Highlander Institute brought local people together from impoverished communities in the Appalachian region to investigate and take action to change their conditions. Describing one meeting at Highlander, Horton recalled the power of local knowledge:

I remember they wanted to know about farm problems. They wanted to know about getting jobs in textile mills. They wanted to know about testing wells for typhoid. We discussed these things. To my amazement my inability to answer questions didn't bother them. . . . That was probably the biggest discovery I ever made. You don't have to know the answers. You raise the questions, sharpen the questions, get people discussing them. And we found that in that group of mountain people a lot of the answers were available if they pooled their knowledge. (Horton 1971, 16–17)

Highlander used a method called "popular education" to empower thousands of community members to collectively tap their own experiences and expertise to change social conditions. Many who attended Highlander, such as Rosa Parks, Ralph Abernathy, and Martin Luther King Jr., would return home to organize for civil, labor, economic, and human rights (Horton 1998).

As McCarthyism lost its sting by the late 1950s and 1960s, academic and social movements questioned previously unchallenged assumptions about science, namely its positivist claims of neutral fact-finding disassociated from social values. In academia, social medicine emerged as a legitimate field of inquiry, reintegrating social science ideas and notions of lay participation into medical research and practice (Porter 1997). The social movements of the 1960s also reengaged local people into the public-health discourse primarily by highlighting that despite rising prosperity and increased access to medical care, inequalities in health persisted for some, particularly for the rural and urban poor.

One example of a civil rights group reconnecting local and professional knowledge for community environmental health is the work of the Young Lords, a group of New York City Puerto Rican activists in El Bario, or East Harlem. The Young Lords organized street cleanups after the sanitation department refused to collect neighborhood garbage for weeks. They convinced local professionals to train them to perform door-to-door lead-poisoning screening and tuberculosis testing (Abramson et al. 1971). The group started day-care programs in local churches, provided breakfast in neighborhood schools, organized tenants to demand housing improvements, and occupied a neighborhood hospital to highlight its inadequate service to the local population. Merging the social, political, and environmental aspects of health, the Young Lords combined local knowledge with professional techniques to address health disparities in their neighborhood (Melendez 2003).

Community mobilizations to address health disparities in the 1960s helped reinvigorate the movement for neighborhood health-centers that had begun fifty years earlier (Schorr and English 1974). Spurred on by the passage of Medicaid and Medicare in 1965 and the Office of Economic Opportunity's Community Action Program (CAP), the neighborhood-health-center movement promoted the health and well-being of impoverished and medically underserved communities by building clinics, developing preventative programs based on team medical practices that involved local people, investigating the environmental causes of poor health, and not limiting their work to categorical disease programs (Hollister et al. 1974). While municipal and state health and welfare departments focused on treating individuals at several locations and departments, neighborhood health centers established "one-stop" locations for clinical and social services, establishing neighborhood institutions run by local people capable of linking existing community resources with newly decentralized governmental programs (Kotler 1969). Neighborhood health centers during this time included the Columbia Point Health Center in a public-housing development in Boston, the Tufts-Delta Health Center in the rural Mound Bayou in the Mississippi Delta, and the North East Neighborhoods Association Health Center in New York City's Lower East Side (Geiger 1967).

During the same time period, a more general public interest in environmental health emerged after a series of highly publicized environmental disasters, such as the contamination of Boston Harbor and the burning Cuyahoga River. These events, combined with the 1962 publication of Rachel Carson's *Silent Spring*, repopularized the nineteenth-century themes of linking industrial pollution and environmental health. The public trust that science was working in the public interest, so dominant in the first half of the twentieth century, had given way to skepticism, citizen action, and calls for new governmental regulations. As Gottlieb notes:

while an earlier critic of the chemical industry, Alice Hamilton, laid the ground-work for discussing environmental themes in an urban-industrial context, Rachel Carson, with the evocative cry in *Silent Spring* . . . brought to the fore questions about the urban and industrial order that a new environmentalism prepared to face. (Gottlieb 1993, 86)

This new environmental activism included community members engaging with and confronting expert views of environmental health hazards, particularly when the hazards were in one's own backyard.

Perhaps the best-known precursor to street science is the grassroots environmental-health activism by residents of Love Canal and of Woburn, Massachusetts. The infamous case at Love Canal, New York, where a concerned mother named Lois Gibbs triggered nationwide interest in the link between landfill contamination and children's health, is the now-classic story of residents organizing to perform and influence science. With the help of Dr. Beverly Paigen, a cancer researcher from Buffalo, Gibbs and other "citizen scientists" were trained to perform telephone and door-to-door health and environmental surveys. This community-driven research found elevated rates of disease but was dismissed by state health officials. Despite the professional rejection of their work, residents pursued, and through the Love Canal Homeowners Association they successfully convinced public officials and scientists to reexamine the environmental health issues in their community. By the summer of 1980 the state and federal government concluded that the neighborhood was unsafe and residents should be relocated.

The Love Canal controversy is an important example of a community struggling to grapple with unexpected health problems because it highlights the challenges local people, public officials, and scientists face when trying to understand the relationships between environmental exposures and health outcomes. Perhaps ironically, the intense scrutiny given to studies of Love Canal residents lead to more rigorous agency peer review, supposedly to ensure the integrity of studies. While at first glance appearing to open up science to public scrutiny, peer review affirmed the proposition that only scientists were qualified to judge the validity of work done by their professional peers. As Jasanoff has noted, self policing not only has enhanced the autonomy and social prestige of science, but it also has encouraged scientists to be accountable to standards considered acceptable by other professionals, not necessarily the general public (1985, 22).

On the heels of the Love Canal controversy another community concerned with sick and dying children, this time in Woburn, Massachusetts,
organized residents to investigate the link between local pollution and illness. The story of Woburn citizens engaging in epidemiologic studies, and
enrolling scientists from Harvard to help them, also is well documented
(Brown and Mikkelsen 1990; Harr 1996). What this case revealed was
that residents with no prior scientific training not only could competently
engage in complex science, but that they had unique information about
exposures and health outcomes that, when combined with traditional epidemiologic methods, could improve scientific inquiry. When a community
organizes to enlist the methods and resources from professional epidemiologists and combines these with insights from residents, they are engaging
in a process Brown and Mikkelsen have called "popular epidemiology"
(1990, 2). When communities engage in science, inject their own knowledge, and reorient investigations, outcomes, and actions, they often are in
the process of seeking environmental health justice.

Environmental-Health Justice and Street Science

The environmental-health-justice movement combines citizen activism
and environmental-health problem solving with demands for civil and
human rights (Bullard 1990; Di Chiro 1998; Cole and Foster 2000).
While this book focuses on one community seeking environmental-
health justice, similar communities around the world are engaging in
street science, often forging research and action partnerships with outsiders, to address the problems they face. A brief review of some of this
work suggests that my study of one neighborhood in Brooklyn is part of
the larger movement for environmental-health justice across the United
States.

In Los Angeles, Communities for a Better Environment (CBE) has
organized poor Latinos to monitor air toxics and address children's
health. Partnering with researchers from the University of California,
CBE activists formed a "bucket brigade" to take street-level air samples,
to analyze these data according to local conditions, and to use these data
to address respiratory-health issues facing local Latino children. These
bucket brigades are groups of local activists that use a low-tech method

for taking air samples "on the street," or where one breathes. CBE has used young people and other community members to take samples of toxic emissions from oil refineries in Contra Costa County. The brigades rely on local knowledge, such as reports of fouls odors, seeing or hearing a release from the plant, and reports of nausea, eye and throat irritation, or other health symptoms, in order to determine when and where to take samples.

In Boston another environmental justice organization, Alternatives for Community and Environment (ACE), is collaborating with professional scientists, including some from the Harvard School of Public Health, to address asthma and air pollution in the Roxbury section of Boston (Loh and Sugerman-Brozan 2002). ACE organized students to map neighborhood land uses and found 15 diesel bus and truck garages within one-half mile of an elementary school. The organization then tapped the knowledge of high-school students to count truck traffic at a neighborhood intersection and identified over 150 diesel vehicles passing through neighborhood streets every hour. Combing the knowledge of young people, their maps, and traffic surveys, ACE partnered with Harvard and the Northeast States for Coordinated Air Use Management to take particulate samples of their own, further documenting the air-pollution problem in their neighborhood. The street science of ACE activists has lead to a state-funded but locally operated comprehensive air-monitoring system, which provides hour-to-hour data on particulate matter pollution over the Web and via telephone.

In San Francisco, the People Organizing to Demand Environmental and Economic Rights or PODER, have organized low-income residents within the Mission District of San Francisco to address environmental, public health, and redevelopment concerns and to help build a land-use agenda within the larger environmental justice movement. As part of their involvement in the Mission Anti-Displacement Coalition, PODER and its members helped develop a grassroots, comprehensive plan for the Mission that was presented to the San Francisco Planning Commission, Planning Department, and Board of Supervisors in July 2003. PODER also has developed a model for EJ groups to partner with one another, and they helped coordinate a report entitled "Building Healthy Communities from the Ground Up: Environmental Justice in California" in coalition with Communities for a Better Environment and the Environmental Health Coalition, another EJ group located in San Diego.

In Albuquerque, New Mexico, the SouthWest Organizing Project (SWOP) and the Southwest Network for Environmental and Economic Justice (SNEEJ), have collaborated with one another to organize residents in Veguita, New Mexico, to address water contamination issues. The organizations trained residents to test their drinking-water wells and perform a community survey of water and illegal-dumping concerns in the South Valley of Albuquerque. This work eventually convinced the U.S. Environmental Protection Agency (EPA) to issue a half-million-dollar grant to the local community and water district to plan, build, and maintain a water-distribution and sanitary-sewer system. SWOP also organized residents to perform air monitoring around the Intel Corporation's Rio Rancho facility as a way to pressure the company to address environmental-health issues for workers and communities along the U.S.-Mexico border. SWOP is a unique EJ group because their partnerships span multiple issues (water and air quality, workers rights, globalization) and multiple constituencies (low-income, Latino/as, youth and elderly, immigrants).

The work of all these groups aims to combine environmental-justice organizing with issues of population health. Each group has forged a collaborative research partnership with one or a host of outside professionals to help them combine community knowledge and experience with professional methods of researching and documenting inequitable environmental-health burdens. When community organizations such as these, and the ones in Brooklyn described in this book, engage in the science of environmental health, they grapple not only with understanding complex environment–human health interactions, but also with how to create more democratic partnerships with scientific and political elites that have traditionally ignored their concerns.

Democracy and Local Knowledge

A fundamental aspect of environmental-health justice is the creation of more democratic partnerships between professionals and the public. This ongoing challenge was perhaps best articulated by John Dewey, in his

1954 work *The Public and Its Problems*, where he highlighted the struggle or "problem" of engaging a citizenry in political processes increasingly dominated by technically elite professionals. Dewey's response was a division of labor; experts would analytically identify problems and citizens would set a democratic agenda for addressing them. The central challenge for Dewey was to devise methods and conditions of public debate, discussion, and persuasion where experts and citizens could integrate their knowledge and understandings. He called for participatory processes to increase the democratic character of decisions, where experts were not asked to judge the efficacy of particular policies, but to act as "interpreters and teachers" to help citizens debate in a way that would reflect the "public interest" (Dewey 1954).

While Dewey's analysis remains important for understanding the democratic challenge presented by street science, his analysis did not fully anticipate the influence of the specialized analyst, operating largely removed from any public discourse, on public policy. Nor did Dewey find the information and knowledge that experts (or lay people for that matter) have problematic; science and expertise for Dewey offered a body of facts and methods that only entered the rhythms and influences of politics at a later stage. Finally, Dewey focused on the optimal procedural conditions for reciprocal dialogue among scientists and lay people, but he did not fully anticipate that the content of the scientist-lay conversation might be problematic; scientists may be unable to translate their information into the ordinary language of everyday practice and publics may be unable to translate their knowledge into the specialized language of science. Thus, the rise of the professional analysts, or technocrat, and an uncritical faith in science as facts and truths, are key components for understanding why professionals tend to ignore community knowledge in environmental-health decision making.

Technocracts, Science, and Local Knowledge

Theda Skocpol, in her book *Civic Engagement in American Democracy*, notes that "today's professionals see themselves as experts who can best contribute to national well being by working with other specialists to tackle complex technical and social problems" (1999, 495). Skocpol continues that these privileged professionals no longer see their role as "working closely with and for non-professional fellow citizens" or help-ing to lead "locally rooted" associations for problem solving. The view that public problems ought to be analyzed by a group of autonomous, highly trained and specialized professionals, who offer their dispassion-ate findings to decision makers, is partially rooted in the belief that facts and values can be separated easily. The positivist view of neutral fact-finding as informing value-laden politics remains a powerful decision-making model in environmental politics (Fischer 2000; Habermas 1970). Perhaps most influential in this view is that one form of rationality has come to dominate environmental politics—where science is the only legitimate form of expertise. Technocrats argue that experience in a given area and training in the specialized collection and systematic analy-sis of information allow them as professionals to tackle issues with neu-trality and dispassionate objectivity (Benveniste 1972).

Yet, political scientists have regularly challenged the technocratic model. For example, Charles Lindblom and David Cohen, in their polemic 1979 book *Usable Knowledge: Social Science and Social Problem Solving,* argue not only that has social policymaking relied too heavily on professionals, but that professional knowledge has not contributed any more than ordinary knowledge to social problem solving. In their strong claim, Lindblom and Cohen (1979) argue for *useable knowledge,* as opposed to the professional knowledge that dominates modern policy-making. The problem with professional knowledge is that it has not deliv-ered on its promise of making better, more efficient, cheaper, more fair or more just social decisions. Nor have the policy sciences contributed a great deal, they argue, to solving some of our most pressing social prob-lems. Lindblom and Cohen (1979) argue for a reintegration of "ordinary knowledge" into policymaking in order to make it more responsive to the needs of the public and to remove the barriers between professional pol-icy makers and citizens.

According to policy analysts like Linblom and Cohen, professionals should not be entrusted to speak for lay publics, especially concerning complex environmental-health controversies. Richard Sclove echoes these concerns in his 1995 book *Democracy and Technology.* Sclove claims that professionals are ill-suited to ensure that science and technol-ogy serve democracy because experts normally are more preoccupied with the mechanisms of science and not its structural bearing on society. Sclove also notes that since "experts enjoy a privileged position within today's inegalitarian political and economic structures, they tend to share with other elites an unstated, and usually quite unconscious, interest in suppressing general awareness of technologies' public, structural face" (1995, 50–51). Additionally, since scientists often have similar backgrounds, professionally socialize, and tend to acquire specialized competence at the expense of integrative knowledge and experience, they are unrepresentative of the "public" and should not be expected to understand or communicate the everyday knowledge of lay people.

Clearly, scientific and technical professionals hold important contributions for environmental-health problem solving, but they alone cannot be expected to ensure science and its results serve the larger society, particularly the least well-off. Lay people often are in a better position than professionals to make judgments over the democratic character of science because they experience how science impacts their everyday lives, from the repetitive mechanical tasks on the factory floor, to navigating inadequate mass-transit systems, to substandard housing and inferior medical care. Thus, to be scientifically and technologically "literate" is to have knowledge and experience not only about a technology's internal principles of operation, but also about how it influences democracy and social justice within the context where it is deployed (Nelkin 1984). Lay people are not only well-situated for this task, they are often more knowledgeable than professionals and therefore ought to be considered "local experts" in their own right.

The Co-Production of Expertise

Since both professionals and lay people have "expert" contributions to make to environmental health decisions, we might think about expertise as being "co-produced." Jasanoff and Wynne (1998) refer to "co-production" to describe the interdependence of scientific knowledge and political order. As mentioned above, in the co-production model, scientific knowledge and social order evolve jointly; science is understood as dependent on the natural world, as well as on historical events, social practices, material resources, and institutions that contribute to the construction, dissemination, and use of scientific knowledge. Political decision making, in the co-production framework, does not take "scientific knowledge" as a given, but seeks to reveal how science is conducted, communicated, and used. The co-production model problematizes knowledge and notions of expertise, challenging hard distinctions between expert and lay ways of knowing. Finally, the co-production model emphasizes that when science is highly uncertain, as in many environmental-health controversies, decisions are inherently "trans-science"—involving questions raised by science but unanswerable by science alone (Weinberg 1972; Jasanoff 1990).

Decision making in the co-production model requires a negotiation among the always partial and plural positions of professionals and lay people (Haraway 1991; Harding 1991). The co-production model also destabilizes the dominant view in science policymaking that science can be uncritically accepted as "fact" and "truth." The destabilizing stories and emphasis on the need for "negotiating expertise" suggest that a deliberative politics is necessary for the co-production of expertise.

In an attempt to articulate how science might be co-produced, Funtowicz and Ravetz call for an "extended peer community" where professionals and publics collaboratively review evidence aimed at improving scientific knowledge:

When problems lack neat solutions, when environmental and ethical aspects of the issues are prominent, when the phenomena themselves are ambiguous, and when all research techniques are open to methodological criticism, then the debates on quality are not enhanced by the exclusion of all but the specialist researchers and official experts. The extension of the peer community is then not merely an ethical or political act; it can possibly *enrich the process of scientific investigation*. (Funtowicz and Ravets 1993, 752–753; emphasis added)

The explicit recognition of both professional information and local knowledge—and that neither ultimately can put to rest the uncertainty of environmental-health problems—can encourage decision makers to acknowledge the necessity of renewal, flexibility, and adjustment as key elements of decision-making success. Instead of portraying themselves as the "source of certainty," professional decision makers can highlight the necessity for contingent decisions that must be open to renegotiation as new information becomes available. This means that the professional's role must be reconceptualized from "guarantor of safety" to "guarantor of recognition"—of new knowledge, new voices, new ideas, new possibilities, and new directions for interventions.

Robert Reich gives an eloquent account of how this practice of public deliberation can spur civic discovery. He suggests that professionals seize the opportunity for the public to deliberate over what it wants by:

convening of various forums . . . where citizens are to discuss whether there is a problem and, if so, what it is and what should be done about it. The public manager does not specifically define the problem or set an objective at the start. . . . Nor does he take formal control of the discussions or determine who should speak for whom. . . . In short, he wants the community to use this as an occasion to debate its future.

Several different kinds of civic discovery may ensue. . . . The problem and its solutions may be redefined. . . . Voluntary action may be generated. . . . Preferences may be legitimized. . . . Individual preferences may be influenced by considerations of what is good for society. . . . Deeper conflicts may be discovered. . . . Deliberation does not automatically generate these public ideas, of course, it simply allows them to arise. Policy making based on interest group intermediation or net benefit maximization, by contrast, offers no such opportunity. (Reich 1988, 144–146)

Both Reich's vision and the process articulated by Funtowicz and Ravetz help frame what the co-production process might look in practice.

However, if co-production requires a negotiation between experts and local people, communities should be weary and enter with caution. As Arnstein's (1969) classic essay on the "ladder of citizen participation" highlighted, public participation can often backfire when the professionals controlling such processes do little to understand the residents of disenfranchised, low-income communities and do even less to meaningfully listen to and include them in decisions. Arnstein wrote that "there is a critical difference between going through the empty ritual of participation and having the real power needed to affect the outcome of the process" (1969, 216).

According to Judith Innes, a professor of urban planning at the University of California, Berkeley, urban planners are attentive to the power dynamics that occur in public dialogues and increasingly "depict planners as embedded in the fabric of community, politics, and public decision-making" (1995, 183). Drawing from critical theory and communicative ethics, this view of planning attempts to ensure, much like Dewey's original problem, that public processes are structured to allow the least powerful, politically disenfranchised to meaningfully participate. In order to accomplish this, a distribution of extra resources, assistance, and guidance to disenfranchised groups by planners may be necessary in order for meaningful and fair public deliberations (Habermas 1984; Forester 1989). The communicative view of planning is employed most often when finding an acceptable policy solution depends on appealing to and mobilizing citizens' knowledge of local or regional conditions, when policy issues have a strong ethical component, and when experts are strongly divided over an issue (Yearley 1999). As planning practitioners are increasingly asked to mediate between professionals and disenfranchised communities in local environmental-health decision making, understanding the benefits and limits of communicative practice becomes a necessary component of the co-production process.

Yet, deliberative forums, especially those involving environmental decisions, rarely have found a way to avoid granting science and technical expertise a privileged position in the discourse (Ozawa and Susskind 1985; Amy 1987). Even some of the most collaborative processes advanced by advocates of consensus building, such as joint fact-finding, have been unable to place science and technical expertise on par with lay knowledge, and these advocates instead recommend not pursuing joint fact-finding when "significant power imbalances among the parties" in a policy dispute exist (Ehrmann and Stinson 1999). Technical language remains a prerequisite for most deliberative forums, often creating an intimidating and "disciplining" barrier for lay citizens seeking to express their disagreements in the language of everyday life (Foucault 1977). Speaking the language of science, as well as the jargon of a particular policy community, remains an essential, but often tacit, credential for participation in environmental health decision making—even in the new deliberative forums. The process of *street science* offers a model for interconnecting and coordinating the different but inherently interdependent discourses of citizens and professionals through the co-production process.

Street Science as a Practice

While traditional policymaking focuses on "problems" and "decisions," deliberative policy science has emphasized *practices* as its unit of analysis (Fischer and Forester 1993). Practice is admittedly a difficult concept.

The concept of practice is an attempt to develop a unified account of knowing and doing (Dewey 1944). Practice emphasizes that knowledge, knowledge application, and knowledge creation cannot be separated from action; knowing and doing are intimately related (Putnam 1995).

This book argues that *street science* is a practice; a practice of science, political inquiry, and action. Street science is not merely a synonym for action. Street science integrates the actor, her resources, and her external environment in one "activity system," in which social, individual, and material aspects are interdependent (Callon 1986; Latour 1993). The focus in such activity systems is on the way the different elements *relate* to each other rather than just on the elements themselves. As Keller and Keller put it:

An individual's knowledge is simultaneously to be regarded as representational and emergent, prepatterned and aimed at coming to terms with actions and products that go beyond the already known. Action has an emergent quality, which results from the continual feedback from external events to internal representations and from the internal representations back to enactment. (Keller and Keller 1993, 127)

Street science in this view acknowledges that the world in which we operate is always to a large extent provisional and improvisational. Action never is controlled completely by the actor, but is influenced by the contingencies of the physical and social world (Putnam 1995).

An important aspect of street science is its social character. Street science originates and evolves in a community—whether community is defined geographically, culturally, or socially. Street science also distances itself from mentalistic and subjectivistic views of judging, assessing, and knowing (Putnam 1995). Street science is a public process that originates and has meaning within a particular community. People learn about the world in shared public processes in which they test what they have learned, often through public discourse.

Central to the communicative dimension of street science are stories. Stories are central to the generative, emergent quality of action in context. Actors negotiate reality by telling *stories* about their own and other people's actions within the various elements of their community. Stories, however, are not merely representations of actions and consequences; stories are generative. As a form of discourse, by telling stories actors simultaneously shape, grasp, and legitimate both their actions and the situation that gave rise to their actions (Throgmorton 1996).

While the co-production model and deliberative practice offer frameworks for how street science might happen, they hardly help with understanding its content. How does local knowledge extend science and improve democracy? The next chapter answers this question by detailing what *local knowledge* means and by showing how it acts as the foundation of the *street science* method of inquiry.

2
Street Science: Characterizing Local Knowledge

Both thinking and facts are changeable, if only because changes in thinking manifest themselves in changed facts. Conversely, fundamental new facts can be discovered only through new thinking.

—Ludwick Fleck, *Genesis and Development of a Scientific Fact*

What is Local Knowledge?

This chapter sets the stage for an analysis of four case studies, in particular outlining what local knowledge is in this context and suggesting how fusing it with expert judgment can form the process of *street science*. As mentioned earlier, scientists and other professionals tend to assume that lay people have little substantive knowledge to offer complex analyses except possibly perceptions and values. This book tends to debunk this idea, beginning here by taking a hard look at the local knowledge offered by community members, distinguishing it from professional knowledge, and highlighting how local knowledge can contribute to complex technical analyses and political decisions.

The policy-sciences literature characterizes local knowledge as "knowledge that does not owe its origin, testing, degree of verification, truth, status, or currency to distinctive . . . professional techniques, but rather to common sense, casual empiricism, or thoughtful speculation and analysis" (Lindblom and Cohen 1979, 12).[6] Local knowledge also includes information pertaining to local contexts or settings, including knowledge of specific characteristics, circumstances, events, and relationships, as well as important understandings of their meaning. A second definition of *local knowledge* comes from Clifford Geertz, whose seminal anthropological work entitled *Local Knowledge* defines it as "practical, collective and strongly rooted in a particular place" that forms an "organized body of thought based on immediacy of experience" (1983, 75). Geertz suggests that local knowledge can be described as simply as "to-know-a-city-is-to-know-its-streets" (1983, 167).[7]

Terminology and language play a particularly important role in discussions of epistemology. For example, studies of international development note that many terms are used to describe what I call local knowledge, including: indigenous knowledge, indigenous technical knowledge, folk knowledge, traditional knowledge, and ethnoecology (Agarwal 1995; Chambers 1997; Irwin 1995; Warren 1991). Each implies something slightly different about how knowledge is "made." For example, Grenier (1998), defines indigenous knowledge as "the unique, traditional, local knowledge existing within and developed around the specific conditions of women and men indigenous to a particular geographic area." The *Indigenous Knowledge and Development Monitor*, an international journal, defines indigenous knowledge as:

The sum total of the knowledge and skills which people in a particular geographic area possess, and which enable them to get the most out of their natural environment. Most of this knowledge and these skills have been passed down from earlier generations, but individual men and women in each new generation adapt and add to this body of knowledge in a constant adjustment to changing circumstances and environmental conditions. They in turn pass on the body of knowledge intact to the next generation, in an effort to provide them with survival strategies.[8]

In the development literature, indigenous knowledge is the preferred term because it implies a *practice* of knowledge-making by certain peoples that occurs through experiential learning rather than a fixed body of information waiting to be acquired in a particular place.

While indigenous may be the most common descriptor used in the development literature, Escobar (1997) and Hobart (1993) note that defining which group or population is indigenous presents a challenge. They suggest that even when indigenousness is measured in terms of prior length of occupancy in a particular place, determinations are never politically neutral, are morally loaded, and inherent ambiguities often elicit more conflict than clarity. Since I am concerned with the knowledge found in Western urban contexts, I have chosen *local* over other possible terms to emphasize the place-based character of this kind of information. *Local* also connotes the situated characteristics and viewpoint associated with knowledge claims and is reflective of the kind of information that urban environmental planners typically find useful (Baum 1997; Fischer 2000). I also chose *local* over other possible descriptors to distinguish it from the nonlocal or removed knowledge produced in settings (e.g., laboratories) where the goal is generalizable universal truths (Latour 1979). Finally, from my vantage point the terms local, indigenous, folk, traditional, etc., often are used interchangeably. Enough overlap among the different definitions exists to ensure a shared intersubjective understanding.

The term *local* comes with it's own historical, moral, and political baggage. For example, local has been associated with particular places, characterized as narrow-minded and parochial, part of a romantic past, an obstacle to modern development and as "a critical component of culturally sensitive modernization" (Agarwal 1995). Local knowledge also might be accused of being moralistic and nationalistic, leading to authoritarian and ethnocentric beliefs that might limit the rights of women and ethnic or religious minorities. Defining local knowledge is far from simple. I will show that the most useful way to understand local knowledge is to reveal how it *differs in practice* from professional ways of knowing and not to romanticize the local as always superior to professional ways of knowing and doing. In addition, I seek to avoid reifying and essentializing local knowledge by suggesting that *local* and *professional* should never be understood as invariant, monolithic, and distinct categories but rather as useful frames for capturing different approaches to knowledge production.

Local and Professional Knowledge

In an effort to avoid essentializing local knowledge by offering one definition, I instead will highlight the particulars in which local and professional knowledge diverge according to the way I am using *local knowledge* in this book. In this vein, I characterize local knowledge in *ideal-type representations* by asking a series of questions about its production. First, I ask who holds local knowledge? This question also might be framed by asking where does local knowledge tend to emerge, both institutionally and culturally? Second, I ask how knowledge is acquired. This question recognizes that lay testing and folk experimentation often underlies local knowledge. In other words, I emphasize that local knowledge is not "mere" belief or a "hunch," but has been subjected to at least common-sense tests of logic, coherence, and rationality that fit with larger community understandings. Third, I ask what makes evidence credible? This question notes that people often measure the credibility of knowledge by whether or not they have actually participated in its production. In the case of environmental hazards, this often means community members conducting *their own* tests with *their own* samples. A fourth question asks in what forums is knowledge tested or legitimated? I acknowledge here that in some public forums, both local and professional knowledge may be competing for legitimacy, such as in the media, so the distinctions between local and professional knowledge may be constantly renegotiated. Finally, I ask what orientation each type of knowledge has toward action. My answers to these questions and the resulting differences between local and professional knowledge are summarized in table 2.1.

While I emphasize key differences between local and other kinds of knowledge, I also note the similarities local knowledge can have with other forms of knowing. In particular, I pay close attention to three potential paradoxes:

a) How to define *local knowledge* while avoiding the tendency to characterize all contextual information as legible to outsiders, thereby potentially emptying local knowledge of its individuality and local variation;

b) How to understand and value knowledge that is specific to a particular place while also trying to grasp its more general appeal (Nelkin 1984);

c) How to define *local knowledge* while acknowledging that all knowledge is to some extent partial, and no single worldview has ultimate access to the "truth" (Shapin 1994).

Examples of Local Knowledge in Environmental Health Policy

I offer three short vignettes of how local, ordinary, or everyday knowledge has been useful in environmental-health decision making. Each sug-

Table 2.1
Local versus Professional Knowledge

Knowledge production question	Local knowledge	Professional knowledge[a]
Who holds it?	Members of community—often identity group/place specific	Members of a profession, university, industry, government agency; sometimes sophisticated NGOs
How is it acquired?	Experience; cultural tradition	Experimental; epidemiologic
What makes evidence credible?	Evidence of one's eyes, lived experience; not instrument-dependent	Highly instrumentally mediated; statistical significance; legal standard
Forums where it is tested?	Public narratives; community stories; courts; media	Peer review; courts; media
Action orientation?[b]	Precautionary/preventative; consensus over causes not necessary	Scientific consensus over causal factors; further study in face of uncertainty

a. By professional knowledge, I am conflating two types of science; research and regulatory. Research science can be thought of as activities aimed at extending knowledge and competence in a particular area without any regard for practical application, while regulatory science consists of activities aimed at improving existing practices, techniques, and processes to further the task of policy development (Jasanoff 1990, 76–77). Jasanoff also notes three different types of scientific activity in regulatory science. First, since regulatory science is sponsored by some entity, it can be thought of as including a component of knowledge production (1990, 77–78). Second, regulatory science involves substantial knowledge synthesis, such as evaluation, screening, and meta-analysis. Third, science intended explicitly for policy involves prediction, such as predicting future risks or costs.

b. There are clear crossovers in this last category, since professional knowledge—holders often hold precautionary views and, likewise, local-knowledge adherents often are perfectly respectful toward professional knowledge and even may think it deserves more deference than their own informal kind of knowing.

gests some of the methods lay people use to gather or shape local knowledge including the importance of local coalitions in knowledge mobilization, how stories and experiences are pooled to create local narratives, how lay people train themselves in science, how they collect and display information, and how local knowledge "travels" into conventional expert domains.

Workers and 2,4,5-T

During discussions of whether the pesticide 2,4,5-T[9] should be banned or regulated in Britain, farm workers challenged experts whose claims of safety ignored the actual conditions and practices workers were subject to when applying the chemical. At the time of the British regulatory debate, a number of other countries already had banned or severely restricted the use of the pesticide. The British National Advisory Committee on Pesticides initially ruled that 2,4,5-T was not harmful to humans when sprayed in calm weather conditions and when workers wore protective clothing and respirators. Farmers were suspicious of the advisory committee's findings, and the farm workers' union organized to testify and offer a combination of its own experience with the pesticide, along with contrary information from established medical sources.

The union gathered testimony on the experiences workers had when using the chemical by distributing a questionnaire, asking about standard chemical application practices and examining health problems that workers or their families were experiencing. Instead of trying to generate statistical data from worker testimony, the union organized the personal accounts into a series of case studies for the advisory committee to review. The workers' stories showed that they were not told about the use restrictions that would make the chemical safe and that they rarely were offered protective clothing or respirators when applying these chemicals. Workers also described the time pressures they were under when applying the chemical, which would prevent them from observing the use-directions prohibiting applying the chemical in conditions such as during high winds and hot weather and in thick undergrowth.

The farm workers' accounts detailed how nonfunctioning or inadequate safety equipment, long distances to washrooms, inadequate cleaning facilities, and lack of proper hazardous-waste disposal, were not merely periodic lapses but normal farm operation. Women working on farms told of numerous miscarriages and birth defects such as cleft palate. The farmers concluded their accounts by suggesting that with the "existence of alternative weed killers and the overall lack of information about the effects on users of 2,4,5-T [under recommended conditions] . . . it became incomprehensible that workers, their families, and the general public would remain subject to these risks" (Irwin 1995, 20).

The farm worker story demonstrated the variability between what the regulators offered as standard operating procedures and the actual conditions surrounding local practices with the chemical, which the farm workers knew from their own experience. The advisory committee reviewed the workers' accounts and concluded that, while compelling, they did not offer statistical evidence showing a causal relationship between worker exposure and health effects. However, the committee members were concerned about the adequacy of the existing regulation, which seemed to be based on false assumptions about pesticide application practices. The stories from the farm workers ignited a debate within the committee that eventually led the commission to reassess the chemical's safety and ban its use in Britain.

Activists and AIDS Research and Policy
The story of AIDS activism in the United States reveals that ordinary people can impact and change the scientific research and decision-making process.[10] From the early 1980s through the mid-1990s, AIDS activists contributed to an understanding of the etiology and treatment of the disease. In reaction to views that the medical community was not addressing the problem of AIDS quickly enough, activists organized and heightened popular resentment against what seemed like recalcitrant scientific experts.

The AIDS movement was organized as a diverse coalition of advocacy organizations, health educators, journalists, artists, and health-service providers. It encompassed the various communities affected most by the AIDS epidemic, including gays, lesbians, hemophiliaes, injection-drug users and members of hard-hit African-American and Latino communities. The movement combined direct-action civil disobedience, such as theatrical attacks on the Food and Drug Administration by the AIDS

Coalition to Unleash Power (ACT-UP), with self-education about the details of virology, immunology, and epidemiology.

Examples of activist influence over AIDS research and policy occurred early on in the history of the disease, when there was substantial debate over what caused it, and later over which therapies "worked." Early scientific thought was that gay promiscuity caused AIDS, but activists challenged this as homophobic speculation. Pressured by both mainstream activists, who began doing their own research on the causes of AIDS, and radical ACT-UP protesters, who galvanized popular sentiment, biomedical researchers looked for other causes and eventually found that a retrovirus was the culprit. After challenging science that seemed to be fueled by antigay lifestyle assumptions, activists also asserted that community-based AIDS organizations had the expertise to define public-health constructs such as "safe sex." As the AIDS epidemic grew in the United States, activists demanded that scientists investigate potentially useful, but risky treatments. After researchers refused, sufferers of the disease learned the science behind their condition and, with no prior experience, took charge of their own experimentation with untested medications. With the help of lay activists who studied how to perform clinical trials, activists conducted their own "underground" drug trials and criticized the methods employed in much AIDS clinical research. The results of the activists trials were made public. With the pressure from activists who won themselves appointments to scientific boards and regulatory review bodies, scientists and regulators were forced to respond.

Over time, through education, use of alternative evidence, and holding a seat at the table with experts, activists began to be acknowledged by the medical and policy community as people who could legitimately speak in the language of medical science, in particular with regard to the design, conduct, and interpretation of clinical trials used to test the safety and efficacy of AIDS drugs. AIDS activists have been successful at provoking lasting changes in how government regulates new drugs and who may participate in the planning and execution of clinical trials. Additionally, the drug "cocktails" that constituted the majority of activist research became the basis of what remains as the most effective treatment for the suppression of AIDS/HIV.

The AIDS activism story is one of credibility struggles regarding whose claims can and should be trusted. It is not about romantic notions of resistance that privileges the "purity" of knowledge seeking from below, but rather a more complicated story of how lay activism influences experts while experts simultaneously transform the practices of the lay people who engage them. The story reveals how citizens can become involved in science and how experts can be forced to find ways to relate to public discourse.

West Harlem and Childhood Asthma

In Harlem, New York, the community organization West Harlem Environmental Action (WEACT) has organized to address one of the nation's highest rates of childhood asthma hospitalizations.[11] Despite alarming rates of asthma, the neighborhood did not have a city-sponsored asthma prevention or research program. WEACT decided to organize youth in the neighborhood to learn more about local respiratory disease risks, to educate youth about how they could reduce their risk of asthma attacks, and to pressure the city, state, and federal governments to address what seemed to be "a growing epidemic."

The WEACT project organized youth to map the assets and hazards, as they saw them, in their neighborhood. A community "risk map" was developed showing areas in the neighborhood where young people experienced foul odors, irritated throats, watery eyes, shortness of breath, and other self-reported symptoms that are known to be precursors of lung dysfunction. The maps also showed assets of the neighborhood, such as parks, stores, and community centers. WEACT and youth activists combined the risk maps with conventional pollution-monitoring information, such as EPA and New York State air-monitoring data, toxic-release-inventory sites, and other noxious facilities. One finding was that many neighborhood youth were hanging out in areas that were in very close proximity to a bus depot, a sewage treatment plant, and a sanitation-truck repair garage.

In an effort to follow up the mapping project, WEACT partnered with the Center for Environmental Health in Northern Manhattan at Columbia University's Mailman School of Public Health. The Columbia University researchers collaborated with youth from WEACT on two studies that examined how air pollution from buses and trucks in West Harlem might be adversely affecting their health. In one study, the partnership obtained data on concentrations of urinary 1-hydroxypyrene (a measure of exposure to polycyclic aromatic hydrocarbons, a component of diesel exhaust) and respiratory and asthma symptoms from seventh-grade students in both an exposed school in West Harlem and a nonexposed school from a sociodemographically similar neighborhood in Central Harlem. The study revealed the specific influence of diesel exhaust on area residents' exposure to fine particles.

In a second study, the youth from WEACT were trained to wear personal air-monitors in order to take air samples at home, at school, and on street corners throughout the neighborhood where they and other youth spent time. The personal monitors gathered measurements of particulates, soluble metals, sulfate, nitrate, and ammonium ions, as well as indoor levels of the pesticide chlordane. Personal air-monitoring was combined with new ambient monitors placed in areas identified as noxious by WEACT, and focused on neighborhood concentrations of volatile organic compounds (VOCs), aldehydes, microscopic particulate matter (PM2.5), and metals. Youth also counted trucks, buses, and cars at the intersections where they wore the monitors. The youth and WEACT staff worked closely with Columbia University scientists to identify the places where monitoring should take place, for how long, at what time of day and season, and how to identify confounding factors such as indoor tobacco smoke. The idea was to try to identify whether specific nodes of pollution exposure for Harlem youth might be contributing to elevated asthma rates and other respiratory disease, and if so, what to do about it. The study, while still ongoing, gathered new air-quality information at the neighborhood level and revealed that West Harlem youth experience significantly elevated exposures to air pollutants at home, at school, and at play.

In both studies, young people had access to information that would have remained inaccessible to scientists. By plotting the location of self-reported respiratory discomfort, WEACT was able to use the youth project to explore possible connections between pollution and health effects. Their hypotheses formed the initial research questions posed by the community organization and the research scientists. The Columbia University scientists helped in legitimating health concerns that WEACT had raised for more than a decade. The cooperative studies kept WEACT activists, both adults and youth, in control of research design, data gathering, and interpreting results—all of which was reflected by the listing of WEACT activists as coauthors in subsequent peer-reviewed publications.

The studies and collaboration between Columbia scientists and WEACT was chosen as a National Institute of Environmental Health Sciences (NIEHS) Highlight of the Month in March of 2000. The research also gained the full financial support from the NIEHS. The studies were presented at U.S. EPA hearings on air-quality standards and played a major role in prompting the agency to propose tighter air-quality standards. The work also highlighted the need for a city-sponsored program to address neighborhood-specific responses to asthma and was instrumental in shaping New York City's first ever Childhood Asthma Initiative (Claudio 2000).

Characterizing Local Knowledge

The three vignettes show how local people—be they workers, health activists, young people, or concerned community members—are more able to deal with complicated social and technical questions than the conventional wisdom generally assumes (Irwin 2001; Wynne 1996). Drawing from these vignettes as well as a review of the literature, the next section of this chapter teases out some specific characteristics of local knowledge by revealing how it contrasts with professional knowledge. I begin from the position that "all knowledge is to some extent both local and partial," in the sense that it comes out of a particular socioeconomic milieu, reflects certain disciplines and training, and depends on certain tools and methods of analysis.

Who Holds Local Knowledge and How Is It Acquired?

Local knowledge often is held by members of a community that can be both geographically located, or place-based, and contextual to specific identity-groups. This means that a "knowledge community" might be a neighborhood and/or a group with a shared culture, symbols, language, religion, norms, or even interests. Specific information about where West Harlem youth hang out is knowledge that only the young people and their trusted peers could provide. The broad coalition built by activists concerned about AIDS is an example of how identity-politics plays an important role in organizing local knowledge.

Knowledge from a particular geographic place simply says, "I live, work, or play here, and therefore I know what is going on." The place aspect of local knowledge stresses that those experiencing disproportionate environmental and disease burdens know more about what these problems mean in their daily lives than anyone else could. The power of place also suggests that those who do not live in these circumstances can never fully understand, so that outsiders must listen carefully to their stories and their ideas (Young 1990). For example, the knowledge of one's geographic place is revealed in the story of an Anniston, Alabama, woman describing a contaminated open-air channel adjacent to her home that carried PCB waste from a neighboring Monsanto plant:

My daughter played in that ditch and my grandbabies, both of them, live on breathing machines. . . . My oldest son played in that ditch. His baby doesn't have any joints in her fingers. . . . It all comes from the chemicals. We live in it all our lives, and this is the result. (Bragg 1997, A16)

Place should be understood as a "material and social space, a *habitus*, infused with different meanings and transected by relations through which particular 'cultural capitals' are formed and transformed" (Healey 1999, 112).[12]

The notion that residents of places and members of groups have a privileged form of expertise about their place and its history and practices is not new to policymaking. It has, however, gained salience in policymaking recently under the guise of the *new social movements* (Calhoun 1994). Identity is understood as constructed socially in relations with others, not taken for granted, and is the social product of the processes by which individuals and groups make sense of the places and situations they face (Giddens 1984). As marginalized groups organize and begin to assign political importance to who they are (i.e., a specific ethnicity or religion) and what they know about their lives (i.e., African-Americans experiencing racism), they often demand that the general public and policy makers respect and acknowledge their self-definitions (Guinier 1994). For these new social movements, identity politics is inherently political because it involves not only seeking recognition, legitimacy, and autonomy, but also refusing, diminishing, and displacing identities others may have assigned. For example, Patricia Collins notes:

By insisting on self-determination, Black women question not only what has been said about African-American women but the credibility and the intentions of those possessing the power to define. When Black women define ourselves, we clearly reject the assumptions that those in positions granting them the authority to interpret our reality are entitled to do so. (Collins 1990, 106–107)

However, this does not mean identity is a fixed concept and predetermined by such things as religion, ethnicity, or neighborhood. The three previous stories make clear that understanding identity means embracing *intersectionality* and *antiessentialism*—or the notions that no person has a single, easily stated, unitary identity, and that no absolute "truth" from any single perspective exists.[13] The AIDS activists came from many identity groups, and activists were as likely to be black Latinas of Caribbean heritage, as they were to be gay, white, heterosexual, Jewish men or suburban housewives with hemophilia. Those who "possess" local knowledge often have conflicting and overlapping identities, loyalties, and allegiances.

The importance of *place* is especially relevant for the work of urban planners. For instance, environmental planners are increasingly acknowledging that place-blind models of decision making are inadequate and have failed to protect some populations (Campbell 1996; Lazarus 1993). Planning is increasingly trying to link decisions to the particulars of the places where decisions are made, as evidenced by such movements as community, equity, and communicative planning (Krumholz and Forester 1990; Forester 1999; Innes 1996). By emphasizing both place and identity, residents with local knowledge might offer planners insight into the different ways that the qualities of places impact on people's sense of well-being. For planners who emphasize place-attentive governance, the task is to identify which social relations really make a difference for improving environmental-health decision making. On the other hand, one danger of emphasizing the place and identity characteristics of local knowledge emerges when such knowledge is "removed" from its context or location. For example, researchers might err if they tried to take the specific insights of monitoring and assessment from Harlem and apply them similarly in all settings of an "urban monitoring" program.

What Makes Evidence Credible
A second aspect of local knowledge is that it rarely conforms to conventional notions of technical rationality, including the need to search for

causal models and reliance on universal principles for getting to the "truth." While I do not want to suggest that local knowledge is always different from scientific or professional ways of knowing, a brief explanation of my understanding of scientific knowledge is needed here in order to explain the differences between expert and local-knowledge approaches to data validation.

Science is a quintessentially public enterprise. Every finding is legitimated by the notion that science is "grounded in impersonal non-private reproducible procedures through which it can be certified by anyone who cares to do so, provided he has the competence and the patience" (Ezrahi 1990, 46). The legitimacy of scientific knowledge often depends on its epistemological differentiation from the everyday knowledge of ordinary people (Shapin 1994). Yet, these boundaries are continually made and remade. Therefore, what is important is to understand how boundaries are made and remade (Gieryn 1995). For instance, disinterested science often portrays itself as apolitical, but its conceptual categories, its rules of evidence, its distinction between appropriate and inappropriate subjects for investigation all reflect the society, and the accompanying social and practical judgments, within which scientists work. Sociologists of science have highlighted the multiplicity, patchiness, and heterogeneity of the space in which scientists work, noting that "expert" science is as much a cultural practice as a rational endeavor (Yearley 1994).

The differences between professional and local ways of knowing can be characterized by examining the emphases each place on information collection methods, standards of evidence, and analytic techniques. Practitioners of local knowledge make explicit their reliance on evidence from time-honored traditions, intuition, images, pictures, oral storytelling, or narratives, as well as visual demonstrations such as street theater. This knowledge is easily accessible to locals and widely shared. Tacit awareness and understanding, which generally are the product of historical experience not merely a hunch, are also explicitly emphasized by practitioners of local knowledge.

In environmental health, community activists often draw from their experiences of seeing or hearing about children with birth defects or from accompanying friends to chemotherapy appointments. At the same time, they observe industry smokestacks and smell the waste-treatment plants in their neighborhoods. Their knowledge comes in part from actual sights, smells, and tastes, the tactile and emotional experiences they encounter in their everyday lives (Tesh 2000). As one community activist stated:

I did not come to the fight against environmental problems as an intellectual but rather as a concerned mother . . . People say, "but you're not a scientist. How do you know it's not safe?" . . . I have common sense . . . I know if dioxin and mercury are going to come out of an incinerator stack, somebody's going to be affected. (Hamilton 1994, 209; ellipses in the original)

Another example of community intuition about environmental-health problems comes from a woman living in Yellow Creek, Kentucky, after the Centers for Disease Control (CDC) found her community's health data statistically insignificant; "Statistics don't tell you. People do. I've walked this creek and I've seen sick people" (Brown and Mikkelson 1990, 129). Although the relationship between industrial chemicals and disease is not something one can just observe or that one can learn by consulting one's body, community activists insist that their intuition, common sense, and experiential knowledge of place gives them privileged insights into local environmental-health problems.

Local people make two very different forms of claims here. The first claim represents a type of local knowledge that *identifies or poses a problem*. This claim is reflected in statements like "I've seen sick people" and highlights contextual knowledge that allows professionals to focus on things they may have missed. Another claim reflects a type of local knowledge that hypothesizes a *relationship between a hazardous exposure and illness*. This claim is reflected in statements such as: "I know if dioxin and mercury are going to come out of an incinerator stack, somebody's going to be affected." Too often professionals assume that local knowledge is only of the second kind, dismiss these claims, and they miss the importance of the first type of local knowledge.

Historically, people's intuition about disease often has changed in response to scientific discoveries. In the early nineteenth century, most physicians believed that the major epidemic diseases were caused by the odor of decaying organic matter. The general public thought so, too, and it seemed entirely reasonable (Rosen 1993). Disease and death rates were lower in rural areas than in urban neighborhoods, where a stench often rose up from piles of rotting kitchen wastes dumped in the streets, from overflowing outhouses behind buildings, and from animal excrement (Melosi 2000). People avoided smells as best they could; common sense told them they caused disease. Later in the century, physicians learned that the smells themselves were not dangerous, but major diseases were caused by microorganisms. Public health officials began spreading this new message to the public and people eventually acquired a "new" understanding of what caused disease (Tesh 1988). They no longer worried about miasmas but about germs and it became "common knowledge" that unwashed hands and bodies as well as imperfectly scrubbed dishes—however clean they might look—could harbor disease-causing bacteria and viruses. Thus, what appears as intuition, especially when it comes to environmental health issues, is often hard to decipher from the images and messages of science, environment, and public health presented by government, corporations, mass media, and public interest groups.

In the 2,4,5-T debate, farm workers claimed a privileged understanding of their health conditions. They constructed narratives about their experience working with the pesticide while the union made a conscious decision not to turn the workers' stories into statistics. Narratives are ways in which people often give meaning to their experiences and events. Oral storytelling is often the medium through which community members express, make sense of, and understand the relationships between their life experiences and the health of their community (Shiva 1997).

Heterogeneity and Hybridity
A third aspect evident from the three vignettes is that local knowledge is not systematized, centralized or static, but constantly renegotiated among those who group it, especially as new circumstances, experiences, and risks emerge in a place. As people reassess new circumstances they reconstruct events and even their own identity, suggesting that local knowledge is fluid and transforming, always partial and imperfect (Haraway 1991). As the AIDS activists learned more about how biomedical research was conducted and as the death rate of AIDS patients soared, activists became more insistent in organizing their own experimental drug trials. Their experiments produced results that were incon-

sistent, but they continued to work to develop a common narrative about the potential utility of experimental drugs. Similarly, the farm workers using 2,4,5-T told different stories about their experience. The union made a conscious effort not to loose this heterogeneity by conflating the narratives into one quantitative assessment. In each case, heterogeneous local knowledge was checked publicly for its validity by, for instance, making test results public and publishing worker's stories.

The qualities of heterogeneity mirror those found in science; definitions of scientific "facts" are constantly open to interpretation and renegotiation (Kuhn 1962). Thus, I am not suggesting a single definition of local knowledge, but rather a heterogeneous, partial, and situated definition, meaning that our varied experiences cause us to see and interpret the world differently (Haraway 1991). Just as no one definition of "expert" or "scientific knowledge" exists today, we should conceptualize local knowledge as a *set* of narratives, tools, and practices located in a particular place, culture, or community.

The narratives of the farm workers using 2,4,5-T suggest that local knowledge does not lend itself easily to precise measurement and quantification. For example, Wynne (1996) describes how Cumbrian sheep farmers' knowledge of soil types was transmitted from practice to practice, not through theory or quantification. The flexibility of relating knowledge to action was evident by the Cumbrian farmers' knowledge of local soil-type variability, since their knowledge of soil types was not constrained by assumptions about standard-type land conditions, but came from grazing experience and noticing how vegetation and soil type changed along the same hillside within the same valley (Wynne 1996). While the characteristics of imprecision and variability might be crucial for the farmer, these same qualities make standardizing and generalizing from local knowledge difficult (Van der Ploeg 1993).

The heterogeneity of local knowledge also suggests that asymmetrical distributions of knowledge exist in a community, often by gender and age, and that no one individual fully "holds it." There also may be disagreements within local accounts, over such things as which stories and evidence count, how they should be appropriated, and who in a community ought to narrate history and make authoritative claims (Agarwal 1995). Further, globalization, mass media, and the Internet have led to a blurring of global-local knowledge distinctions. Any definition today of "local" surely will be influenced by, for example, conventional standards of scientific proof (Shiva 2000). Again, the more I attempt to demarcate the boundaries between local and professional knowledge, the more the dichotomy becomes blurry and the contextual nature of "expertise" becomes evident.

Oppositional Discourse
A fourth characteristic of those who rely on local knowledge is that their information is confrontational, although not necessarily antagonistic, to conventional science and expertise (Agarwal 1995; Gaventa 1993). Knowledge claims are always embedded in power relationships (Foucault 1977). Power is expressed in public decision making by who gets to define problems, offer evidence, be heard, and design solutions. Professional knowledge currently retains hegemony over these features of environmental-health research and decision making. Yet, those who hold local knowledge offer counter stories which can displace, challenge, or simply mock the dominant discourse. Local knowledge offers what Nancy Fraser (1992) has called an "oppositional discourse" much like, for example, feminist discourse. The farm workers using 2,4,5-T, WEACT, and AIDS activists all were attempting to confront experts who either were ignoring their situation or, in the activists' eyes, not generating relevant knowledge that would help solve their particular problems.

Importantly, what the AIDS and WEACT activists' accounts revealed is that confrontations with expert and scientific knowledge can occur when activists try and stake out part of the scientists' terrain. This claim is fundamentally different from activists who simply distrust experts and always view them with suspicion, from those who claim science and truth are on their side because they have hired their own experts, and from those who outright reject the scientific way of knowing and advance claims to expertise based on a wholly different epistemological standpoint (Nelkin 1995). Confrontation occurs, for example, when the AIDS and WEACT activists wrangle with scientists about issues of truth and method, exerting pressure on them from both the outside and locating themselves on the "inside" of research. These activists challenge not just the use and control of science and expert knowledge, but also the content and processes by which knowledge is produced. Fundamentally, these activists claim to speak credibly as experts in their own right, as people who know about things scientific and who can partake of this special and powerful discourse of truth. When the holders of local knowledge confront experts by offering their own evidence and by trying to change the rules of who is qualified to play the game of knowledge making from both inside and outside the field, they not only are confronting, but also are *doing* science (Irwin 1995).

Finally, the narratives describing local knowledge often cause confrontation by giving voice to the often-silent suffering of disadvantaged people. The sharing of stories and personal narratives can demonstrate that others have similar experiences. This was evident to the union as they gathered stories from the farm workers using 2,4,5-T. In order to confront dominant discourses, local people often have to carry a "double consciousness" of both conventional and local knowledge (Du Bois 1990; Andersen 1999). In *The Souls of Black Folk* (1990), Du Bois described a double consciousness in black Americans, a dual lens through which the dialectic of black self-recognition was of being in America but not of it. When black Americans faced the burden of trying to be accepted in white culture, Du Bois notes they lived "a double life, with double thoughts, double duties, and double social classes . . . giving rise to double words and double ideals, and tempt the mind to pretence or to revolt, to hypocrisy or to radicalism" (1990, 146). When the holders of local knowledge attempt to be heard in the realm of professionals, they must manage the tension of valuing their own experiences while simulataneously accepting the worldview of professionals. As Du Bois noted: "It is a peculiar sensation, this double-consciousness, this sense of always looking at one's self through the eyes of others, of measuring one's soul by the tape of a world that looks on in amused contempt and pity" (1990, 8). Since community members often will carry the double burden of "translating" their knowledge into language professionals can understand, they must be "multilingual" in both their own and the dominant discourse. This double burden presents a challenge for the successful sharing of community knowledge in professional decision-making forums.

Challenges to the Professional Uptake of Local Knowledge

The previous section highlighted why local knowledge is different from professional knowledge and why local knowledge is a useful category at all. It also described the major contrasts between professional and local knowledge. This section explores how community members can insert their local knowledge into environmental policymaking and the challenges facing its uptake in professional decision-making circles.

Highlighting Discreditable/Inaccurate Expert Knowledge
The knowledge of local people often is revealed, especially to those outside the local community, when locals sense that expert analyses or decision making has inaccurately portrayed their experience. The farm workers using 2,4,5-T gathered stories describing "standard" practice in response to what they felt were inaccurate expert assumptions. Similarly, the AIDS activists did not believe that biomedical researchers and the governmental institutions supporting them were acting quickly enough or in the interest of dying victims. The WEACT activists also did not believe that environmental regulators were doing enough both to monitor and to prevent air pollution or asthma in their neighborhood. These activists took action because they believed that the institutions entrusted to protect them had failed.

Wynne (1996) suggests that public response to experts often has as much to do with the complexities of the issue at hand as with the historical relationships the public or particular groups have with the institutions offering the technical information. In other words, local knowledge often is revealed because of, for instance, a lack of local trust in the social institutions performing assessments or making difficult decisions. The activists revealed that a corollary to trust is *control*. The AIDS and WEACT activists confronted experts in part to gain control over their own situation.

Truth claims in science emerge because scientists either trust that an experiment was competently performed (thus granting credibility to the results) or they trust the result (thereby conceding that the experiment was competently performed). At any given moment, *some* knowledge must be taken on faith if science is to proceed. Even distrust is predicated on a background of trust; a scientist cannot distrust a particular finding or person except against a background of other shared knowledge which is unproblematically trusted (Shapin 1994, 17).

Trust and credibility are fragile in the scientific community and are highly guarded through such mechanisms as allocating research funds, judging other's work, and policing abuses (Jasanoff 1990). But for lay people, trust in experts must be found through external markers of credibility such as the institutional affiliations of researchers, their source of funding, where findings are published and, possibly, what the *New York Times* says about the findings. Having lay people challenge the credibility, legitimacy, and trustworthiness of experts can be very threatening for professionals, since their resources and maintenance of professional autonomy may be placed in jeopardy. When the local knowledge of community people enters environmental-health problem solving, the normal flow of trust and credibility between expert institutions and lay people is disrupted. Thus, when lay people offer local knowledge about problematic situations, they might highlight experts' inaccuracies and simultaneously disrupt the taken-for-granted trust and credibility the public confers on expert institutions.

Extending the Work of Professionals
While local knowledge often can be revealed in response to the inaccurate work of experts, it can simultaneously contribute to the experts' work. By challenging entrenched expert paradigms of problem definition and analysis, holders of local knowledge attempt to revalue forms of knowledge that professional science has excluded. For example, the AIDS and WEACT activists engaged with scientists to make professionals and public policy respond to their concerns. Both sets of activists also provided expert researchers with access to data and information that they could not have known easily in the absence of local participation. Those who advocate for local knowledge in environmental-health decision making often seek to reorient understandings gained from conventional science, rather than to dismiss professional findings outright. Usually community members focus on aspects of problem solving that tend to be neglected in traditional accounts of scientific practice: uncertainty, social values, and a plurality of legitimate perspectives.

Policy analysts regularly document how science transforms society (Ezrahi 1990; Jasanoff 1996). Less often appreciated is how society, by speaking back to experts, can transform science and accompanying decision making.[14] When lay people "speak back" to experts and science, one thing they do is contextualize science by attempting to make it "work" and resonate with their lived experience (Gibbons 1999). This process most often occurs when scientists, administrators, and lay people deliberate over controversial environmental choices. It also can occur when local people are allowed to interpret scientific understandings through their own experiences. When lay people bring science that historically had remained in the lab into their daily lives, the information and knowledge of science must now be valid in both the laboratory and "on the street"—demanding what Gibbons (1999) has called "socially robust knowledge." Ideally, socially robust knowledge achieves validity through an extended group of experts, including "lay experts," where different representations of knowledge are negotiated for their relevance to particular on-the-ground problems (Funtowicz and Ravetz 1993). The implication is a shift from science "speaking truth" to society, to the socially robust notion of "making sense together" (O'Neill 1974; Schutz 1976).[15]

While local knowledge often can extend the work of conventional science, the legitimacy of local knowledge should not be discounted if it does not fit neatly into the categories of conventional science. Legitimizing local knowledge only when the holders of local knowledge can extend the work of experts would lead to a situation in which local knowledge is judged according to universalistic scientific standards instead of on its contextual merits. This tension currently is being played out in the debate over intellectual-property rights, where agricultural and pharmaceutical companies have sought to codify and exploit local knowledge for commercial purposes. In some cases, corporate scientists enter communities to learn the time-tested healing traditions of an Amazonian tribe or the farming techniques of an Andean village, then upon their return to the North, sell these techniques and patent them as their own proprietary knowledge (Shiva 1997). While a full discussion of intellectual-property rights and local knowledge is beyond the scope of this chapter, the example is raised here to highlight how insights from local knowledge can both extend the work of experts and simultaneously be removed, disassociated, and exploited from its origins, often at the expense of those who developed and shared it in the first place (Shiva 2000).

Reorienting Problematic Situations

Practitioners of local knowledge also can influence environmental-health decision making when they go beyond description to offer analytic and prescriptive advice. In reorienting problematic situations, locals might attempt to redefine accepted social conditions, define what is just, and even assign responsibility for perceived injustice. The farm workers using 2,4,5-T were successful in using their experiential knowledge of working conditions to redefine "standard practice" and reorient the way decision makers viewed the efficacy of safety measures associated with the application of the pesticide. The worker narratives altered systems of belief and typical categories by calling attention to neglected evidence.

When community activists in environmental-health decision making use local knowledge to reframe a problem offered by experts, local activists attempt to make problems align with their particular "capital"—or their form of credibility—in order to have a say in problem solving (Bourdieu 1977). In public decision making, power often is manifested in the ability of professionals to label, classify, and condemn, as well as in the capacity of publics to resist the imposition of certain expert definitions (Foucault 1977). In "reframing" problems, holders of local knowledge can "create value" by identifying additional considerations and options for action unseen by others.[16]

The notion of policy framing often is used to described how ideas become practice (Goffman 1971; Schon and Rein 1994). Frames impose order upon experience. For example, diseases often have been framed through attributions of causality and blame, leading to what seems like inevitable social action (Rosenberg 1992). Similarly, Jasanoff (1990) notes how scientific advisory boards often frame environmental-risk questions and conflate science evidence with social and political judgments.

Schon (1983) highlights the importance of policy framing for both professionals and lay publics. According to Schon, a lack of authentic expert-client interaction in policy sciences exists, and one consequence is an adherence to the technical model of rationality and the subordination of the client by professionals. This subordination of the client, or lay citizen, has given rise to one-dimensional, distorted communications between practitioners and clients, ultimately impeding the activity most crucial for effective practice, what Schon (1983) calls "problem setting." In problem setting, analyses focus on identification and discovery, a "conversation with the situation," and often require the consensual reshaping of new problem orientations in order to determine (a) relevant problem situations to be addressed, and (b) the theoretical normative frames that structure and shape our basic understandings of (and discourses about) particular policy issues, including evaluation criteria. Schon (1983) describes problem setting as preceding technical problem solving and calls for "reflection in action" where practitioners and lay people in dialogue with one another set the problem-solving agenda.

Suggesting Precautionary and Contingent Action

Local knowledge also can be used to influence decision making by highlighting preventative, precautionary, and contingent actions. The farm workers using 2,4,5-T made explicit in their statement to the Advisory Committee that with the existence of alternative pesticides and the uncertainty and lack of information about the effects of 2,4,5-T on workers, the regulatory body should opt for caution and not take the risk of exposing anyone to potential risks from the pesticide. The AIDS activists were not necessarily precautionary, but they advocated for contingent action, pressuring scientists and policy makers to approve experimental drugs until new information revealed that the treatments were ineffective or harmful, or another safer and more effective treatment was discovered.

Communities of disadvantaged populations who suffer from disease or environmental exposures often recognize that environmental-health decision making must proceed under a veil of uncertainty. These populations cannot wait for "definitive proof" to guide interventions and commonly invoke the "precautionary principle" when acting on local information. The precautionary principle states that "when an activity raises threats of harm to human health and the environment, precautionary measures should be taken even if some cause-effect relationships are not fully established scientifically" (Raffensperger and Tickner 1999, 24). When communities invoke the precautionary principle, they are demanding that preventative and anticipatory action be taken, that the burden for proof of safety be placed on the proponent of a potentially harmful activity, that safer alternatives to the potential harm be explored, and that those asked to live with a potential harm be democratically involved in scientific decision making.

The Contributions of Local Knowledge to Environmental Health Policy

This chapter has shown that local knowledge is important in its own right. I also argue in this book that local knowledge improves environmental-health research and policy making, and I will show how local knowledge helps do this in at least four ways:

(a) *Epistemology*   local knowledge makes a cognitive contribution by rectifying the tendency toward reductionism in professional vision and policy;

(b) *Procedural Democracy*   local knowledge contributes additional and previously excluded voices, which can promote wider acceptance of decisions by fostering a "hybridizing" of professional discourse with local experience;

(c) *Effectiveness*   local knowledge can point out low-cost and more efficient intervention options;

(d) *Distributive Justice*   local knowledge can raise previously unacknowledged *distributive justice* concerns facing disadvantaged communities.

The *epistemology* category can be factored out into four additional subcategories:

(i) *Aggregation*   that is, professional decision-making tools always aggregate, and this misses local particularity;

(ii) *Heterogeneity*   local knowledge can highlight how professional assessment models pay inadequate heed to the inter-individual or inter-group variability of the population on which the model is being imposed;

(iii) *Lifestyle*   professional models always try to say something about the relevant causal factors, and in so doing, they necessarily bound some things out as not relevant. From the community perspective, this condition says "your professional model of how I'm going to react (my body or my community) to this exposure is flawed because you are not taking a holistic enough look at how I move through the world";

(iv) *Tacit Knowledge*   local knowledge reveals the unspoken information that does not easily lend itself to the reductionist model-making that is characteristic of professional science.

Epistemology

The first category posits that local knowledge can make a contribution to the knowledge base used for environmental-health research and policy making. Part of the knowledge base for environmental-health decisions comes from professional science, or information emerging from a profession or discipline that undergoes a series of professional legitimacy "tests" (i.e., case-controlled experiments, statistical analyses, peer review, etc.). On the other hand, local knowledge can be thought of as deriving less from professional techniques and more from time-honored sources such as intuition, images, pictures, oral storytelling or narratives, and visual demonstrations, and is "tested" via public dialogues and storytelling. The epistemological category looks at how local people engage with and seek to extend science, but do not outright reject science. When lay people work to extend science with their own knowledge, they change the ground rules about how science is conducted.[17] An example of lay people working to extend science is the practice of "popular epidemiology" described in this book's introduction. By entering the domain of professional science, lay people seek "to re-value forms of knowledge that professional science has excluded, rather than to devalue scientific knowledge itself" (Cozzens and Woodhouse 1995, 538). When lay people attempt to extend science, they expand the circle of participation, create value by identifying additional considerations, challenge professional methods as inadequate representations of the sum total of reality, and fundamentally alter the existing rules of the "scientific field."[18] At least four subcategories help clarify how local knowledge extends science.

Aggregation   Aggregation suggests that professional decision-making tools always form a singular whole, tending to miss local particularity. Local knowledge can point out where an insupportable degree of aggregation is taking place. As I will show in the air toxics and mapping case, community members pointed out to the EPA that its dispersion modeling of air toxics in the community missed small emission sources, and in particular, potentially dangerous perchloroethylene emissions from dry cleaners located in residential buildings. Thus, the aggregation category suggests that an epistemological flaw occurs when professional methods of data aggregation do not look at individual sources or particularities within the community, and this flaw can be corrected through local knowledge.

Heterogeneity   The heterogeneity category suggests that professional models of hazards pay inadequate heed to the heterogeneity of population groups on which the model is being imposed. Inter-individual or inter-group variability is revealed by local knowledge when, for instance, women and young people are asked questions and considered serious sources of information about asthma, as described in chapter 4. Heterogeneity also says that African-Americans, Latinos, Slavic immigrants, and Hasidic Jews do not have the same diet, and this was an important insight from community members when the EPA assumed an "urban default diet" when assessing dietary exposures, as described in chapter 3. The heterogeneity of a population, which local knowledge can expose, is critically important for understanding inter-individual and inter-group susceptibility to certain hazardous exposures, such as different diets, because such things as body weight, lung development in children, lead consumption, etc., all play a role in making some individuals/groups more susceptible to the same hazardous exposure. Yet, the heterogeneity of a population often is washed-out when professional models treat all population groups the same.

Lifestyles   The lifestyle category says that since professional models are always trying to say something about the relevant causal factors, they necessarily bound some things out as not relevant. Local knowledge captures the information that is often ruled out by professionals as "a way of living." For example, chapter 3 shows that the practices of urban anglers were not apparent to the EPA, but even if they had been, urban fishing likely would have been treated as a lifestyle issue and not relevant to human-health-risk assessment. This analytic category suggests that professional scientists tend to overlook the fact that local people with particular lifestyles can be good sources of information about technical matters. For instance, Bruno Latour (1988) notes in his "science in action" framework—which reveals that how scientists construct their workday, their networks of colleagues, and their lobbying in the outside world all shape their definition of what is acceptable science—that the real meaning of epidemiological "facts" cannot be understood until the professional experiences the problem in its community setting. When residents in New York's Greenpoint/Williamsburg neighborhood tell professionals that they need to pay attention to lifestyle factors, as Latinos did when discussing the use of herbal home remedies (chapter 4), they are saying that the professional model is inadequate because it has bounded out of its cognitive domain things that do affect health and illness. Local knowledge demands that professional models look more holistically at how community residents are living. The lifestyles category is not merely saying "you have to give weight to me and my experience" as a narrative voice, but rather it says "your professional model of how I'm going to react (my body or my community) to this exposure is flawed because you are not taking a holistic enough look at how I move through the world." This dynamic also is clear in chapter 5 when, after the City finds no risk to locals from the sand blasting of lead paint, residents claim that the City's study doesn't reflect their experience because it didn't use local soil, resident's own blood, or actual lead measurements in the community. In other words, residents failed to "see themselves" in the science, and the professional study failed to bring on board the very public whose health it was trying to assess.

Tacit Knowledge   The tacit knowledge category says that local knowledge truthfully can discover information that does not lend itself easily to the reductionist model-making characteristic of professional science. The most obvious example of this occurs when professionals do research on the mafia; they can't get truthful information unless they become part of the community, and some information is so tacit that only members of the community can gather it. We will see examples of this in chapter 4, when residents attempt a community-wide asthma survey and find out that Hasidic community members are uncomfortable talking with outsiders. The Hasidim only are willing to perform asthma research with their own people. Another example is in chapter 3, when gathering information about anglers is performed by community members with whom anglers share common language, cultural heritage, socioeconomic background, and immigration status—all counteracting disincentives and allaying fears for anglers' participation in research. Tacit knowledge is like the "hidden transcripts" of community members, constructed by locals without outsider awareness of their existence or content (Scott 1990). However, when hidden transcripts are publicly revealed, dominated groups can offer insights unknowable to outsiders and can contribute to new understandings that might change structural power relations.

Procedural Democracy This category claims that local knowledge improves procedural democracy by including previously excluded and marginalized voices—in a world where expertise tends to exclude people. Procedural democracy entails the right to treatment with equal concern and respect in political decisions about how goods and opportunities are to be distributed, and focuses on the fairness of decision making. Including local knowledge with professional science can foster a "hybridizing" of professional discourse with local experience and ultimately promote wider democratic legitimacy for professional decisions. This category explores whether democracy is enhanced when the voices of local knowledge are included into professional policy discourse.

Effectiveness The effectiveness category claims that local knowledge can help identify low-cost policy options and more efficiently target intervention strategies. Low-cost policy options might include community residents' performing education or information dissemination themselves. By including local knowledge in professional science, community members are more likely to "see themselves" in science, thus finding it more acceptable and potentially saving time and money in policymaking. Implementation of policy options is likely to be more effective when local knowledge highlights existing practices embedded in the community that might affect an intervention, such as the cultural medicinal practices of Latinos discussed in chapter 4.

Distributive Justice   Local knowledge can highlight distributive justice concerns of community residents. Distributive justice is the right to the same distribution of goods and opportunities as anyone has or is given. In environmental health terms, it refers to the disproportionate public-health and environmental hazards, and lack of environmental benefits (i.e., parks, sewerage, safe drinking water, public transportation, etc.), borne by people of color and those with lower incomes. For instance, as seen in chapter 3, residents were concerned with asking whether the risk assessment captured the potentially hazardous diets of anglers, a particular subpopulation in the community. Chapter 6 recounts residents challenging the EPA air-toxic model for missing hazards in homes above dry cleaners. In both instances, local knowledge asks "who are the persons at risk," not just what level of risk is ultimately acceptable.

This chapter has outlined why local knowledge is a useful category, its differences with professional knowledge, some of the challenges facing its uptake by professional decision makers, and how it is useful in policymaking by contributing both epistemologically and normatively to environmental-health decision making. Local knowledge has authority beyond the often assumed parochial, subjective, and emotional world of the community members who hold it. Local knowledge also has problematized our conventional understanding of professional knowledge, particularly questioning the dichotomy between professional and lay expertise. The porous boundaries between local and professional knowledge suggests that planners and policy makers interested in democratic practice ought to pay attention to local knowledge as they manage processes that legitimate some information as relevant for decision making.

This, however, calls for new practices and professional-local relationships. These practices must find new ways of expanding the knowledge base and fusing local and professional knowledge, not on deciding which alternative—professional or local—is best. The next four chapters present more detailed studies of how local and professional knowledge might be fused—how *street science* operates in practice—in order to improve environmental-health decision making.

3

Risk Assessment, Community Knowledge, and Subsistence Anglers

On any morning they are out there, steady as the sun rise. Along the pier at India Street and the vacant lot off Kent Avenue, the fisherman line up every morning. I love coming out here because it is my time to ease into the day . . . you know have a smoke, coffee, watch the traffic build on the FDR in the city. I mean you can't beat this view of Manhattan! For some of these guys, boy, it ain't a hobby. They got the system down: a few different rods, nets, tackle boxes, the whole 'nine. Know what I mean? They're back here in the afternoons. For me its fun, but its also dinner sometimes.

—Carlos, describing the action along the East River in Greenpoint/Williamsburg on a typical morning, June 3, 2000

This chapter shows how the knowledge of community residents improved environmental-health decision making in Greenpoint/Williamsburg (G/W). The story reveals how residents of G/W, organized by the Watchperson Project, gathered information about subsistence angler practices and how these data were used to improve the EPA's Cumulative Exposure Project in the neighborhood. Information about subsistence anglers was a type of local knowledge that only members of the community could truthfully collect. This information eventually was incorporated into the EPA assessment and improved both professional and local understanding of the hazards facing community residents living off subsistence diets of locally caught fish.

The Cumulative Exposure Project

In 1995, the EPA was considering using its newly devised program for modeling air toxics at the community level. The agency had developed a model for estimating the dispersion of air toxics at the census-tract level nationwide. The methodology allowed regulators, for the first time, to estimate the concentration of 148 hazardous air pollutants (HAPs) at a small scale—an aggregation at which air pollutants are suspected of impacting human health. Before the development of the national air-toxics modeling project, HAPs were either measured pollutant-by-pollutant, or they were not measured at all. The development of the air-toxic dispersion model allowed the agency to consider assessing the human-health and environmental impacts of multiple toxins at a very fine scale.

The air-toxic modeling formed the centerpiece of a new program at the EPA called the Cumulative Exposure Project (CEP). The intent of CEP was to combine air-toxic modeling with similar multitoxin inputs for other ingestion pathways, such as through food and drinking water, and to derive a cumulative-exposure profile for states, regions, and even neighborhoods. The CEP represented a new movement within EPA for looking at alternatives to traditional risk-assessment techniques, a movement which is questioning the assumptions behind the use and methods of risk assessment (EPA 2004; Finkel and Golding 1994).

For most of its history, the EPA has assessed risks and made environmental-protection decisions based on individual contaminants—such as lead, chlordane, and DDT—with risk assessments for these chemicals often focused on one source, pathway, or adverse effect. In 1997, the EPA announced guidance for cumulative assessments, which they claimed would allow them to describe and quantify the risks that Americans face from many sources of pollution, rather than by one pollutant at a time. According to the memorandum by then–EPA administrator Carol Browner:

We are increasingly able to assess not simply whether a population is at risk, but how that risk presents itself. In addition, we are better able in many cases to analyze risks by considering any unique impacts the risks may elicit due to the gender, ethnicity, geographic origin, or age of the affected populations. Where data are available, therefore, we may be able to determine more precisely whether environmental threats pose a greater risk to women, children, the elderly, and other specific populations, and whether a cumulative exposure to many contaminants, in combination, poses a greater risk to the public. (EPA 1997)

This shift at the EPA occurred in large part because of criticisms of risk assessment by environmental justice (EJ) activists and their sympathetic academic supporters (Goldman 2000; Sexton 2000). The EJ movement had been arguing for a shift away from risk assessment because it saw the process as systematically burdening those populations that were already disproportionately exposed: the poor and people of color. EJ activists argued that when risk assessment relied on a single exposure pathway, source, and health endpoint (with an almost exclusive emphasis on carcinogenesis), it ignored the multiple pathways, numerous sources of toxic exposures, and noncancer health endpoints that disproportionately afflict poor populations and people of color (Gibbs 1994). The activists also challenged risk assessment because the process had become so complex that it became the exclusive domain of highly specialized experts. The result, claimed EJ activists, was an expert-dominated process that excluded the very populations that assessments were supposed to protect.

The exclusivity of the risk-assessment process was a critique echoed by other environmental and public-health reformers who sought to challenge the EPA's risk-analysis framework more generally. The risk-analysis framework separated the assessment, management, and communication of risks into three distinct and independent processes. In this scheme technical experts performed the assessments, which were supposed to inform policy administrators, who made risk management decisions, which were then "communicated" to concerned publics by a third set of administrative specialists. Both the reformers and EJ activists pressured the EPA throughout the 1990s to "democratize" the analysis process by, among other things, including those being asked to bear risks in the assessment itself. They also were pressuring the EPA to move away from the conventional risk-assessment process toward alternative hazard-assessment and decision-making processes such as comparative risk analysis and cumulative risk assessment (NRC 1996).

At the same time the EPA was exploring methods for cumulative assessments, the New York City (NYC) Department of Environmental Protection (DEP) also was working on a project to measure the cumulative environmental burdens in city neighborhoods. The DEP had initiated the Baseline Aggregate Environmental Load (BAEL, pronounced "bail") project (Osleeb et al. 1997). The BAEL project was part of the Environmental Benefits Program (EBP) at the DEP (Sweeney et al. 1994). The agency was forced to establish the EBP after community groups pressured New York State to enforce Clean Water Act violations by the DEP at the Newtown Creek sewage treatment plant in Greenpoint. The state ordered the DEP to fund a Supplemental Environmental Program, and the EBP was one result (ICLEI 1993). It was during EBP meetings with community groups, including the Watchperson Project (now funded as part of the EBP), that the BAEL project was conceptualized (Cooper 1995).

The BAEL project attempted to derive a weighted measure for the cumulative environmental burden for each city block in New York City. This was clearly a mammoth undertaking, but its first tasks were to gather as much existing environmental data available for the G/W community and place this into a database that could be joined with the City's database of every land parcel. The idea was to develop an "environmental load" profile for each land parcel in G/W based on zoning, land use, and existing environmental data (Osleeb et al. 1997). The DEP also enrolled the U.S. EPA in this effort to help with data analysis.

While the BAEL and EPA projects proceeded, residents of G/W organized to stop the siting and operation of additional noxious facilities. Residents had organized to stop an incinerator from operating in the neighborhood and had organized to stop the siting of two garbage-transfer stations. The community argued that the garbage-transfer stations violated environmental and health regulations when the two new projects were considered in combination with the other existing twenty-eight transfer stations in the neighborhood. The cumulative effects, the community argued, represented a blatant violation of the EPA's commitment to environmental justice, and the community called on the U.S. Department of Justice (DOJ) to hold a hearing. At the hearing in G/W, the EPA was asked to explain its position on cumulative risk (Martin 1998b; Shin 1999).

At the request of local and national environmental-justice activists, the EPA responded to the hearing and the BAEL project by deciding to pilot the cumulative-exposure project in G/W.[19] According to the EPA, G/W had the three elements that could lead to a successful pilot project: an active and organized citizenry, available local and national data, and the presence of many hazards suggesting that the agency was "likely to find something" (Talcott 1999).

The EPA chose to develop its research methodology for the CEP in consultation with its consultant, Industrial Economics, Inc. of Cambridge, Massachusetts, and the NYC DEP, but not with the community. At the urging of the DEP's Director of the EBP, Eva Hanhardt, the EPA did present their methodology at a community meeting. Having been party to the BAEL discussions, the activists were fairly well versed in cumulative assessments and immediately noted some gaps in the EPA's proposed methodology, such as its inattention to small source polluters (Hanhardt 1999). One of the activists' particular concerns was that the EPA proposal made no mention of assessing potentially toxic exposures from eating fish caught in the neighboring East River.

The EPA food-exposure assessment included information on the average Northeast "urban diet" from the National Health and Nutrition Examination Survey, but the survey made no mention of diets that might consist of locally caught fish. EPA scientists were surprised to hear from community members that residents were eating fish from the East River (Talcott 1999). The EPA had no data to confirm or dispute this claim. The activists, specifically the Watchperson Project, offered to gather some information on local anglers to show EPA that it was a serious issue. At first the EPA refused. They were intent on using their proposed method, which assessed food exposures using exposure estimates based on the typical urban diet in the Northeastern United States. The Watchperson Project argued that without the angler information, CEP would miss an important potentially hazardous exposure. The community group also noted that the anglers would be unlikely to talk with outsiders about their practices because many of the anglers were immigrants and non-English speakers who ate the fish because of both poverty and cultural tradition. The group argued that only local people could gather this important information. While these arguments seemed persuasive, it was only after the EPA visited the community and the Watchperson Project staff took them on a tour of the piers along the East River that the agency acquiesced and agreed to let the community organization interview anglers (Swanston 2000; Hanhardt 1999).

The EPA chose to work with the Watchperson Project to devise an interview protocol and methods for collecting information. The Watchperson Project enlisted volunteers to interview local anglers and collect information on subsistence fish diets in the neighborhood. The group gathered stories of anglers and collected survey data. The remainder of this chapter explores in more detail the processes the Watchperson Project used to collect information from the anglers. It shows how the activities of local activists revealed how local knowledge can improve professional decision making by:

(a) Adding data sources such as angler information;

(b) Providing access to difficult to reach informants, such as immigrants;

(c) Bridging linguistic differences, by relying on non-English speakers; and

(d) Counteracting disincentives of informants to participate, due to poverty, culture, fear and defensiveness.

It also reveals how the community-gathered information influenced EPA. But first, a review of the EJ movement's critique of the conventional risk-assessment process is important for understanding how and why the EPA's CEP emerged in Greenpoint/Williamsburg originally.

Professional Views of Risk Assessment

The conventional process for assessing hazards in a community involves quantitative risk assessment. This process has remained relatively the same since the first EPA guidance memorandum on the topic was issued in the early 1980s (NRC 1983). In risk assessment, one identifies an environmental hazard, describes the potential adverse effects on a hypothetical individual exposed to that hazard, and estimates the probability of an adverse effect to a hypothetical individual (EPA 1986). The process includes identifying a single hazard, evaluating how much of the hazard—the dose—stimulates an adverse response, and estimating how often and at what concentrations humans are exposed to the hazard. These three steps—hazard identification, dose-response, and exposure assessment—are combined into the fourth step, generating a risk characterization (NRC 1983).

Hazard identification is a process whereby analysts use available evidence to determine whether a substance is linked to a particular human-health or environmental effect (Wilson and Crouch 1987; Kammen and Hassenzahl 1999). This generally involves EPA scientists reviewing respected health studies to determine whether a chemical or other substance poses a threat to human health. Researchers typically use data from long-term animal bioassays (Wildavsky and Levenson 1995). EPA generally chooses a uniform, or default, set of assumptions from these studies, which are then applied to each substance assessed (Paustenbach 1989). Risk assessors use these judgments as the default toxicity weightings for chemicals they are studying (Graham and Wiener 1995).

The second step in risk assessment, dose-response, is a way to estimate the relationship between exposure to a harmful substance and its potential effects on health. Data on the human health effects due to exposure are in short supply, largely because most experimenting on humans is unethical, so dose-response assessment typically requires researchers to employ sophisticated mathematical techniques to extrapolate effects that could occur in humans who are exposed at low doses from data on health effects observed in rodents that were given relatively high doses (Wildavsky and Levenson 1995). Such techniques rely on low-dose-extrapolation models (Kammen and Hassenzahl 1999). Of the four risk assessment steps, dose-response assessment may contain the most uncertainty. Whether the effects observed in animals administered high doses can be extrapolated to accurately reflect what people encounter in their everyday environment is difficult to know. In attempts to be extraconservative regarding carcinogenesis, the EPA recommends using a "linearized multistage" (LMS) model, meaning that scientists assume that increased dosage of a substance will lead to increased incidence of cancer and that there is no threshold level (i.e., all nonzero doses have some positive effect) (Paustenbach 1989). In the end, the methods employed in low-dose extrapolation must use complicated statistical models and not biological information, suggesting that the dose-response function is more a statistical measurement than a real estimator of disease (Ozonoff and Boden 1987).

Exposure assessment is the third stage of a risk assessment. At this stage, analysts attempt to identify what proportion of a population will receive some exposure to a substance. Exposure assessment methods can vary greatly, depending on the type of pollution source. For example, the exposure assessment for dispersion of air pollution bears little resemblance to the exposure assessment for the dispersion of pollutants from a landfill (Kammen and Hassenzahl 1999). Relevant data for exposure assessment consist of information that is usually well known or readily knowable—the concentration of a chemical at a pollution source, the nature of migration from the source, and the location of the surrounding people (Wilson and Crouch 1987). The difficulties arise in choosing a concentration (i.e., daily, monthly, yearly averages) to model key fate and transport assumptions (i.e., meteorological data) and which receptors to include (i.e., what distance from source, sensitive populations, treat all people the same).

Risk characterization is the fourth and final stage of a traditional quantitative risk assessment. Multiplying the harm from incremental doses (the number derived from the dose-response assessment) by the dose a population is expected to receive (the number derived from the exposure assessment) generates the risk characterization (Kammen and Hassenzahl 1999). The resulting number is supposed to represent the threat to a population from the concentration of a chemical that might reach them. However, the risk characterization merely consists of a "stacking" of all the uncertainties of the exposure assessment with all the uncertainties of the dose-response function (Ozonoff and Boden 1987). This process can mask the uncertainties in the previous steps, thereby inaccurately portraying the potential severity of the risk.

By emphasizing the scientific objectivity of the procedure, risk assessment tries to offer policy makers a means to persuade the public that regulatory decisions are based on rational analysis (Jasanoff 1990). One intention of risk assessment is to enhance public confidence in the impartiality of regulatory agencies decisions. While the models and default assumptions used for site-specific risk assessments are intended to protect public health, many scientists and risk-assessment professionals state that the subjective judgments inherent in risk assessment make the process more art than science, and its weaknesses are "an open secret" (Lash

1994). In fact, William Ruckelshaus, a former EPA administrator, once described risk assessment data as "like the captured spy: If you torture it long enough it will tell you anything you want to know" (Ruckelshaus 1984, 158).

Environmental-justice activists have offered some specific challenges to the risk-assessment process. First, they claim that the process focuses on individual contaminants from one source—with an overwhelming emphasis on carcinogenisis—while ignoring the multiple hazards that usually face low-income populations and communities of color (Kuehn 1996). Second, activists claim that the institutionalized risk discourse, which requires descriptions of hazards to be made in quantitative terms in the categories of the four-stage assessment process, has systematically excluded lay knowledge and observations from the assessment and decision-making process. The process has ignored lay judgments by creating hard boundaries between what counts as scientific expertise and what is relegated to merely political values (Bryant 1995; Collin and Collin 1998; Di Chiro 1998).

Community Challenges to Risk Assessment: Procedural and Distributive Justice

Quantitative risk assessments rarely distinguish inter-individual variability in susceptibility to disease. The default assumption generally employed in risk assessment is that humans on average have the same susceptibility as persons in epidemiological studies or as the most sensitive of the animal species tested (EPA 1986). However, Zahm et al. (1994) report that in a survey of occupational-cancer epidemiological studies, only *two percent* of the studies included any analysis of the effects on nonwhite women, and only *seven percent* addressed the effects on nonwhite men. King (1996) notes the persistent underrepresentation of nonwhites in epidemiological studies, clinical trials, and medical textbooks. The EPA default "reference man" for developing dose-response predictions has been described as "a seventy-kilogram man with the general biology of a Caucasian" (Kuehn 1996). While EPA acknowledged in its 1992 *Environmental Equity Report* that health risks differ according to race and class, the agency continues to rely on the default dose-response assumptions that all humans are equally exposed and susceptible for risk-assessment purposes (EPA 1992). The present practice of excluding information regarding the hazards faced by more susceptible ethnic and racial subpopulations results in an assessment that fails to reflect higher environmental risks to those groups.

A second challenge states that traditional risk assessment fails to account for how *discrimination* might influence health. Epidemiologists have been studying how being treated as a second-class citizen—based on economic status, ethnicity, gender, disability, and age—influences health for over a century and a half (Krieger and Fee 1996; Porter 1997). However, new areas of epidemiology such as "ecosocial theory" take the notion of "embodiment" literally and highlight how we literally incorporate biologically—from conception to death—our social experiences and express this embodiment in population patterns of health, disease, and well-being (Krieger 2000). This theory explicitly recognizes the social, economic, and political judgments that help produce population distributions of health, including: (a) societal arrangements of power and property, and contingent patterns of production and consumption, and (b) constraints and possibilities of our biology, as shaped by our species' evolutionary history, our ecologic context, and individual trajectories of biological and social development (Krieger 2001). Together these factors structure inequalities in exposure and susceptibility to—and potentially options for resisting—pathogenic insults and processes across populations.

A third critique suggests that risk assessment's almost exclusive focus on cancer ignores important noncancer health effects, such as respiratory, neurologic, reproductive, and psychological disorders (Kuehn 1996). Overreliance on cancer leaves many other serious diseases and human-health problems unaddressed—many of which appear to disproportionately afflict low-income communities and people of color (NIH 2004; NIEHS 2004; Geronimous 2000). Even when cancer acts as the primary focus for risk assessment, environmental-justice critics note that assessments only identify single exposures from a single source. Cumulative exposures, where individuals are exposed to numerous chemicals through different media and/or sources, are rarely if ever part of a risk assessment (NRC 1996).

One reason cumulative risk is not considered in traditional risk assessment is that the exposures individuals experience before the addition of a new exposure—referred to as the "background exposure" condition—are rarely known. The importance of this information becomes apparent when questions of chemical additivity and synergism are considered. *Chemical additivity* occurs when chemicals or pollutants mix and result in an exact combination of all their individual effects (i.e., a chemical with a toxicity of two plus another chemical with a toxicity of two might result in a mixture with a toxicity of four). *Synergism* occurs when chemicals combine for a greater additive effect (i.e., toxicity of two plus toxicity of two results in a toxicity of ten). Conversely, *antagonism* of chemicals can occur, where the combined result is a diminished toxicity. Yet, since toxicology has not developed an accepted method for determining these effects, they are ignored in traditional risk assessment (Kammen and Hassenzahl 1999).

Since people of color and low-income communities face greater exposures to environmental contaminants, the failure of risk assessment to account for multiple and cumulative exposures may be harming these subpopulations greatest. The 1992 EPA report on *Environmental Equity* and the 1999 Institute of Medicine report *Toward Environmental Justice* both state that racial and ethnic minority groups and low-income populations have greater-than-average observed exposures to pollutants because of where they live, where they work, and what they consume (EPA 1992; IOM 1999). The higher exposures experienced by these communities mean that risk assessment's failure to take account of cumulative and multiple exposures and its failure to aggregate risks based on race, ethnicity, and class, result in risk characterizations that are less accurate for low-income populations and people of color.

Finally, communities criticize risk assessment because it tends to rely on quantitative data over the experiences of those living with persistent pollution (Collin and Collin 1998; Di Chiro 1998). Quantitative analysis often leads to what Tribe called the "dwarfing of soft variables": information that cannot be quantified is not considered, and conclusions are biased toward considerations that the quantification process can incorporate (Tribe 1972). Environmental-justice advocates are often more concerned with asking *who* are the persons at risk rather than, for example, whether one-in-a-million is an acceptable level of risk (Bullard and Johnson 2000). While risk implies that the chance of the harm in question is accepted willingly in the expectation of gain, many environmental-justice activists are concerned about whether those who bear the harm will actually receive any of the gains and if risks can be eliminated entirely. By engaging in debates over risk calculations, the discourse of environmental policy is shifted from talk of hazards and dangers to the notion of "risk" that implies that the chance of harm in question *is accepted willingly* with the expectation of some gain (Winner 1986). O'Brien (2000) suggests that before risk is selected as a focus in any area of policy discussion, other available ways of defining the question should be thoroughly investigated, since the initial definition of the problem shapes who is empowered to dictate the conversation and who will be excluded, deemed inarticulate, irrelevant, or incompetent. Lois Gibbs characterizes risk assessment as describing the "risks that someone else has chosen for you to take" (Gibbs 1994, 329).

Despite these critiques, risk assessment continues to drive environmental-health decision making and to demarcate who is "expert" to make judgments over potentially hazardous situations. For example, U.S. Supreme Court Chief Justice Stephen Breyer has called for bureaucratically rational risk assessment to be insulated from politics and the public in a federal "superagency" assigned all risk-assessment duties (Breyer 1993). However, the EPA, the Science Advisory Board, the National Research Council, and the Presidential/Congressional Commission on Risk Assessment and Management all have rejected Breyer's suggestion; they instead recommend meaningful public input in all stages of hazard assessments (SAB 1999; PCRARM 1997). According to the 1996 National Research Council report, *Understanding Risk: Informing Decisions in a Democratic Society*, a new assessment process should include constant public feedback, so that initial problem frames can be revisited and redrawn in the light of new information and experiences. The report noted the following advantages of public participation in the process (SAB 1999, 30):

• Clarifying and potentially advancing resolution of issues of fairness. (When we use the word "fairness" we are referring to both distributional and procedural equity, two issues that have been concerns of the Environmental Justice movement.)

• Informing multi-dimensional tradeoffs among efficiency, fairness, environmental sustainability and other concerns.

• Increasing credibility.

• Informing priorities for research. Studies suggest that more data are not necessarily better for organizational decision-making. Deliberation can help determine the research that is most likely to be key to decision-making.

The SAB also noted that making ever-smaller reductions in selected single risks may not be the best policy either for protecting overall environmental quality or for making the best use of society's resources (SAB 1999, 5). Finally, the EPA's cumulative-risk-assessment guidance states that the agency's goal is to ensure that citizens and other stakeholders have an opportunity to help define the way in which an environmental or public-health problem is assessed, to understand how the available data are used in the risk assessment, and to see how the data affect decisions about risk management (EPA 1997). In this context, and in response to the challenges raised by environmental-justice activists, the EPA initiated its Cumulative Exposure Project in the Greenpoint/Williamsburg neighborhood.

The Cumulative Exposure Project in Greeenpoint/Williamsburg

The CEP began in 1994 as an EPA pilot study to model exposures to hazardous air pollutants nationwide, a mandate given the EPA in the 1990 Clean Air Act (EPA 2000). The air toxics assessment was intended to help states identify and prioritize those air toxics that might present the greatest potential health risks and those with the highest concentrations for regulatory purposes. Building on prior EPA work on integrated risk assessments, the CEP aimed at moving beyond the source-by-source approach to human-health risk assessment by recognizing that populations are simultaneously exposed to multiple environmental pollutants from multiple sources (Woodruff et al. 1998). It attempts this in two ways: by summing up the combination of chemicals in a community's environment, and by translating this information into a cumulative risk profile (EPA 2001). CEP sought to combine the modeling of air toxic exposure with multiple pollutant exposures from other media, such as water and food, in order to identify communities or demographic groups most at risk (EPA 2001).

Cumulative assessments are intended to differ from the single-source risk assessment approach on a number of fronts (table 3.1). EPA's Guidance on Cumulative Risk Assessment states:

The practice of risk assessment within the Environmental Protection Agency is evolving away from a focus on the potential of a single pollutant in one environmental medium for causing cancer toward integrated assessments involving suites of pollutants in several media that may cause a variety of adverse effects on humans, plants, animals, or even effects on ecological systems and their processes and functions. (EPA 1997, ii)

Cumulative assessments consider multiple pathways, sources, and endpoints, while conventional risk assessments only consider a single pathway, source, and endpoint (EPA 1997). For example, exposure assessment focuses on populations, not individuals, and aggregates by population subgroups, such as those highly exposed and highly sensitive. Highly exposed populations are further aggregated by specific geographic area (i.e., neighborhoods), age, gender, race, ethnicity, and economic status, while highly sensitive populations are aggregated by such categories as those with preexisting conditions (i.e., asthmatics), age (i.e., infants), and gender (i.e., pregnant women). Cumulative assessments also focus on multiple pathways, such as ingestion, inhalation, and dermal contact, while also looking for potential routes of community exposure, such as direct or indirect contact, bioaccumulation, biomagnification, and vector transfers (i.e., mosquito bites). Since the focus is on exposures, multiple human-health endpoints—carcinogenic, neurotoxicologic, reproductive, developmental, immunologic, renal, hepatic, etc.—are considered. While conventional risk assessment models a linear acute dose of a toxin, cumulative exposure assessment considers the different frequencies, durations, and intensities of exposures, such as chronic low doses without any observable adverse effect. Finally, the EPA claims that cumulative assessments shift the process from the conventional "one-size-fits-all" centralized model of decision making to a case-specific, community-based

Table 3.1
Risk Assessment versus Cumulative Exposure Assessment

Traditional risk assessment	Cumulative exposure assessment
Single exposure pathway	Ingestion, inhalation, dermal, and indirect
Single source	Multiple sources
Single endpoint (carcinogenesis)	Exposures not single disease
One linear dose (mostly high acute)	Varied dosage (includes low-chronic)
Modeling (dependent on rodent studies)	Epidemiological and no-observed-effects considered
Maximally exposed individual	Actual measured exposures
Probability outcome—point or Monte Carlo	Characterization by toxicity and health endpoints
One-size-fits-all, single stressor	Case-specific, holistic
Expert-dominated, centralized assessment	Community-based decision making

Source: U.S. EPA. Cumulative Risk Assessment Guidance. Science Policy Council. Available: http://www.epa.gov/ORD/spc/2cumrisk.htm.

decision-making model (CEQ 1996; EPA 1997).

The CEP uses existing data and methods to evaluate exposures through three different pathways—air, food, and drinking water. The food component aimed to estimate exposures to 37 contaminants in 34 different foods (EPA 2001). The original proposal by the EPA was to analyze food-exposure levels across the entire community population and then aggregate the analysis by age subgroups (EPA 1999a). Contaminants of concern consisted of pesticide residues and common industrial pollutants found in produce, meats, and dairy products. The analysis combined data on contaminant concentrations in specific foods with data on patterns of consumption, mostly derived from default values estimated for a typical urban diet (EPA 1999a). The aim was to generate a set of estimates of average daily-contaminant exposures summed across different types of food (Talcott 1999). To evaluate the significance of these estimated exposures, the estimates are compared to toxicity values for each contaminant. According to the EPA's CEP guidance documents the analytic methodology used to estimate the average toxic exposures from food involves four separate steps (EPA 1999a):

1) Creating a food contaminant database by obtaining and compiling measured contaminant data;

2) Creating a food consumption data base that provides information on consumption patterns by population subgroup;

3) Combining contaminant and consumption information to estimate exposures from individual food types; and

4) Estimating total dietary exposures by summing across all food types.

The EPA methodology called for calculations of exposures for each food identified as common to the population, and these estimates then would be summed across different food types and for each contaminant (EPA 1999a).

Local Contributions to the Dietary Exposure Assessment

While developing the methodology for and gathering data on neighborhood exposures, the EPA relied on its own experts, consultants, and the NYC DEP for some neighborhood environmental-monitoring data. The EPA had no definitive plan for public participation while conducting the project in G/W (Talcott 1999). However, at the request of the then-EBP-director Eva Hanhardt, the EPA scheduled a series of community meetings to inform the community about the CEP and to ensure the agency was capturing as many potentially hazardous environmental exposures as possible. The DEP already was working with many of the community organizations on the BAEL project and sensed that the EPA project would be entirely rejected if the agency did not consult with residents (Hanhardt 2000).

During the first community meeting, the agency heard from residents that the existing data were a good first step but, according to Samara Swanston, Director of the Watchperson Project, insufficient to characterize the multiple hazards in the neighborhood (Swanston 2000). In particular, residents noted that the EPA's approach for assessing dietary risks was based on a series of default "urban diet" assumptions, which lacked any specific information about the potential hazards from eating locally caught fish. According to Swanston:

When we heard they were going to assess dietary risks using some default diet, we all just rolled our eyes. You've got Hasidic Jews here eating only kosher; Poles eating an Eastern European diet; Puerto Ricans, Dominicans and Guyanese. I mean it is like the UN of food over here. You're gonna tell this community we've got an "average American" diet?

For many residents, the EPA's assumption of an "urban default diet" represented a lack of sensitivity to local culture and further stirred mistrust. According to Swanston:

At the meeting we finally got EPA to let us review their research protocol. The thing that jumped out to us was the culturally insensitive language, like not recognizing that people of color do not have choices about where they could live. The language was also insensitive to cultural tradition and it sounded like they were blaming us for fishing from the river. The use of default assumptions really raised skepticism that the project was going to do anything more than just rubber-stamp what community members already knew; that we are a highly exposed community. A little thing like the wrong assumptions about what people eat had most people associate the EPA project with another wasted effort by government on a study that was going to sit on a shelf somewhere and not help anyone.

According to Fred Talcott (1999) of the EPA, the agency knew of the local ethnic diversity but was unsure how this might influence their assessment of dietary risks: "In the absence of information on the eating habits of these ethnic groups, we chose to use the default assumptions. We didn't anticipate that this would raise such a red-flag with the community."

Residents suggested during the meeting that a large number of local people were living off a diet of fish caught from the East River. This was the first time the EPA had heard of this potential health hazard. According to one EPA official:

When the residents raised the concern about people fishing out the East River we initially responded by saying, "we understand recreational fishing can pose a health risk, but we do not think the practice of eating fish is that widespread." But, the residents insisted that this was not a recreational activity; many families were eating fish from the river as a staple of their diet. To be honest, we were in disbelief and shocked.[20]

While the EPA was skeptical of the community's concerns, in part because residents only had anecdotal evidence about the extent of local subsistence-fish diets, the agency also knew that if the claims were true they presented a potentially serious toxic exposure for local people.

Hazards from Urban Fish Diets

Of all the risks facing the poor and people of color, the health hazards from eating toxic fish may be the least understood and given the least attention (IOM 1999). The EPA and Institute of Medicine both have recognized that subsistence-fish diets represent a real and potentially significant source of contamination for the urban poor, immigrants, and people of color (EPA 1992; IOM 1999). However, understanding the potential health risks from subsistence fish diets of urban populations has proved difficult, since researchers rarely gather these data or monitor the dietary practices of urban populations (West et al. 1995). These data are also difficult to gather. For example, a study of NYC anglers found that they are reluctant to participate in studies because they are immigrants, are not comfortable having their traditional practices studied, and are non-English speakers (Burger, Staine, and Gochfeld 1993). Researchers have recognized, however, that food, and fish in particular, is integral to the cultural identity and even the survival of some urban populations (EPA 1999b).

The EPA has recognized that sociocultural considerations are important when assessing fish consumption, especially for new immigrants since food habits are some of the most resistant to change (EPA 1999b). Food habits often act to maintain cultural identity, particularly for those groups for whom the consumption of fish is a long-standing tradition. The EPA report notes:

Fish, as an important cultural resource, may contribute to community well-being and cohesiveness . . . may hold a prominent place in religious and cultural rituals . . . [and] often involves the intergenerational transfer of knowledge and may contribute to sharing and social bonding within family and community. For some, the consumption of self-caught fish is an important means of augmenting family food supplies; it has important economic impacts. (EPA 1999b, 5-1)

Other researchers have noted that fish foods among immigrants serve as a link to the past, ease the shock of entering a new culture, and provide a means to maintain ethnic identity (Story and Harris 1989). When strong cultural ties are linked to fish diets, it may be difficult for these populations to conceive of these foods as hazardous, particularly if immediate negative health effects are not perceived to occur (EPA 1999b, 5-2).

The most common contaminants found in fish include chlordane, chlorpyrifos, polychlorinated biphenols (PCBs), DDT, methyl mercury (MeHg), and other pesticides and industrial chemicals discharged in surface waters from nonpoint sources (EPA 1999b).[21] Heavy metals commonly found in fish, such as cadmium and lead, have been linked to immunosuppression, which is suspected of causing decreased resistance to infections. Schantz et al. (2001) note that impairments of memory and learning can occur from consuming fish contaminated with PCBs. The EPA warns that intake of PCBs from fish has been associated with liver disease, diabetes, compromised immune function, thyroid effects, and increased cancer risks, particularly non-Hodgkins lymphoma. Methyl mercury, a neurotoxin, presents a risk for brain and nervous system damage, especially to children and unborn babies of mothers who eat mercury-contaminated fish during pregnancy. The EPA recommends that women who are pregnant or may become pregnant, nursing mothers, and young children limit their consumption of fish caught by family and friends to one meal per week. PCBs and mercury are particularly dangerous to subsistence anglers because the concentrations of these toxins tend to build up, or *bioaccumulate*, in fish and human-fatty tissue, and they do not degrade or disappear like some other persistent organic pollutants (EPA 1999b).

The Knowledge of Anglers Contributing to Professional Knowledge

The EPA faced a dilemma with regard to the neighborhood anglers. They knew eating locally caught fish presented a potential toxic exposure, but they had no data regarding this exposure. The Watchperson Project, volunteering to interview local anglers and collect data that potentially could be used in the exposure assessment, emphasized to EPA that since many of the anglers were immigrants and non-English speakers, the locals would be reluctant to speak with outside researchers. According to Swanston of the Watchperson Project:

After we took the EPA people on a trip to the piers, it was clear to them that there were a lot of locals eating fish from the river. They also saw that almost none of the fisherman were speaking English or even looked like most of the EPA people. If they wanted information about who was eating fish, I think it was obvious to them that community people—African-Americans, Spanish and Polish speakers—were going to have to collect the data. The fishermen were not going to talk to some government officials. Not around here. (Swanston 2000)

The tour of the community was a significant event for convincing the EPA about the seriousness of the problem and whose claims should and can be trusted and who was credible to gather additional information. Community-lead tours, often called "toxic tours," are rituals of learning. Forester (1999) notes that these rituals are performances that enable learning, by both locals and outsiders.

We can think of participatory rituals as encounters that enable participants to develop more familiar relationships or to learn more about one another before solving the problems they face—for example, the informal drink before negotiations; the meals during focused workshops. . . . Participatory rituals are encounters in which "meeting those people" comes first, even if it serves the secondary objective of "solving our problem." On such occasions we discover that we learn about our problems through, and as we learn about, other participants too. (Forester 1999, 131–132).

Thus, local knowledge is not just about providing information, but involves professionals' participation in rituals that allow residents to gather local data.

After considering whether to ignore the subsistence-fishing exposures altogether or have community members gather this information, EPA agreed to help the Watchperson Project collect information about the practices of local anglers. According to Talcott of the EPA:

After the tour and learning from residents that they were eating fish from the East River, we had no choice but to let the community groups gather the data. For a number of reasons, including language, cultural barriers and potential trust issues, we felt the local people could best gather this data. This was one situation where residents raised an issue we hadn't considered, defined the extent of the problem, and provided the data for analysis.

The Watchperson Project developed a protocol for interviewing anglers to identify approximately how many people were eating fish out of the river, the amounts and frequency of fish consumption, and the types of fish anglers and their families were eating (Swanston 2000). With the help of EPA survey instruments used to capture similar information in other communities, the Watchperson Project tailored a survey for the local population (EPA 1993, 1994, 1999a). According to Swanston:

The EPA and their consultants gave us lots of ideas and sample surveys and these were useful for asking some questions. But, at the end of the day, we had a good sense of what to ask and how to ask it. A lot of the language of the questionnaires the EPA people gave us had no sensitivity to Black or Latino culture. They gave us surveys from the Midwest or Alaska, or ones for Native Americans. Most of the language and questions were either Euro-centric or not really relevant for people in this community. (Swanston 2000)

The community group spent ten weeks interviewing anglers at the India Street and the North Seventh Street/Kent Street piers along the East River. Community members volunteering with the Watchperson Project visited the piers twice a day for two weeks during August and September and observed and interviewed over 200 anglers. Each angler was asked about age, race, country of origin, and the number and ages of people in their family. The species of fish and the number they regularly caught was also reviewed. Since the interviewing was conducted during the summer, each interview included questions about seasonal variability and frequency of catches in different seasons. Finally, each angler was asked about her or his fish consumption patterns and those of the family, including the species, quantities, and preparation techniques of the fish they ate (Swanston 2000; EPA 1999a).

Some Angler Stories
Along with administering and collecting survey data, the Watchperson Project interviewed anglers to get a better sense of why they might be eating fish from the river, and whether the anglers thought there was a health risk for themselves or their families from eating the fish. The interviews provided the stories or narratives behind the anglers' practices.[22] While the Watchperson Project did not systematically record the interviews, they informally recounted what they heard from anglers for the EPA when they presented their survey findings.

Jose and Ricardo,[23] a Puerto Rican and Dominican both in their "late forties," spoke about why they fished from the river and whether they thought there was a potential health problem. Their account was typical of most anglers in the G/W community.

Jose: My Dad used to take me fishing in *Fajardo* [a coastal area in Puerto Rico] and those were the best times of my youth. I mean doing a family-type thing; how could that be unsafe, right?

Ricardo: The cops don't bother us down here and fishin' keeps me outta trouble. I mean don't got no body breathin' down your neck out here.

J: Yeah, *mira*, at home [Dominican Republic] eating fish was for survival. Really, it ain't much different for us here. I got to feed myself and three kids and every fish I catch is one less thing we got to buy.

R: The fish we catch are fresher, you know, than anywhere else. I know the government people put up signs once in a while to say stop fishing or something. I'm not really sure what the signs say and within a few days some homeless guy's tore it down for firewood anyway.

J: We ain't stupid, we know this river isn't the cleanest. It is probably polluted. I mean I wouldn't swim in here or nothin'. But this cove over here, it's pretty clean. There ain't no dead fish. Its not so bad. And, the fish we catch come in from the Atlantic, they don't feed in here. So, they don't got no chemicals in them. I mean we don't know anyone whose gotten sick from eating what we catch here.

R: We've been out here a long time. I was taught how to recognize a bad one [fish]; you look for lesions, make sure it is the right color and if it smells funny, we throw it back. You can smell the bad ones usually.

J: Yeah, you know we clean and cook 'em real good too. That is the best way to make them safe. If I thought there was a problem, I wouldn't be feeding these fish to my kids a few times a week. My family depends on me for food. My neighbors even buy my catch sometimes. They trust me. I know a clean catch.

Stories like these suggested to the Watchperson Project and the EPA that many anglers were eating fish from the East River both because it was part of their cultural tradition and a way to survive. They also imply that anglers have a sense that some fish might be contaminated ("the river isn't the cleanest"), but that somehow the fish they are catching and eating are safe ("this cove is clean"; "the fish we catch come in from the Atlantic"). The anglers also told interviewers that they would know when a fish was contaminated through visual inspections or smell ("I was taught to recognize bad ones"; "it is the right color"; "you can smell the bad ones"). Finally, subsistence anglers typically believed that the fish they were feeding their families with was safe because of the way they cooked and cleaned the fish. Interviews like these were important. They provided the narratives or stories that helped make sense of and provide contextual meanings to the survey data.

Angler Survey Findings

The community-gathered information was divided by age and ethnicity, and separate categories were created for whites, Poles, African-Americans, and Latinos. Almost all the anglers interviewed were Latino or African-American, although some were Caucasian (primarily Slavic). Of the Latinos, most had origins in Puerto Rico, the Dominican Republic, or Ecuador (Swanston 2000). The Watchperson Project also found that almost all the anglers were males between the ages of 16 and 60. The anglers' family sizes ranged from 3 to 10 persons, and all anglers interviewed noted that at least 1 family member was under the age of 19. The Watchperson Project survey determined that local anglers were catching between 40 and 75 fish per week, averaging 57 fish per week, and that each family member of an angler was eating approximately 9.5 local fish per week (EPA 1999a).

During the survey, each angler was asked to identify the four species they most frequently caught and consumed. All the anglers interviewed listed the same four species: blue crab, American eel, blue fish, and striped bass (EPA 1999a). Most anglers reported that they ate whatever they caught. One of the challenges for the interviewers was that anglers might not have been identifying the fish they caught and ate accurately (Swanston 2000). Therefore, the interviewers also collected fish samples to confirm species identification.

During the Watchperson Project's surveying and interviewing, EPA analysts met with the community group several times to determine whether subsistence fishing really constituted the potential risk residents claimed. The EPA emphasized that the meetings were to help the group organize its findings in a useable way. The EPA did not, however, interfere with the data collection; this was left entirely to the community group. The interviewers' stories played a role in convincing the EPA about the prevalence of local subsistence anglers and the potential severity of the risks facing hundreds of residents. According to one EPA analyst:

We were never quite sure the community survey was going to be helpful or that eating local fish was really that big of an issue. But then we started to hear how many people the community group was talking to, their ethnicity and the sheer amount of fish they were catching. The preliminary accounts were compelling and surprising to many of us. We started to believe this was a potentially serious issue in the community. That's when we realized that good data on the anglers would be important to complete the exposure assessment.

After compiling the data they collected, the Watchperson Project met with EPA analysts to present the information. According to Swanston, by the time of the meeting the EPA officials seemed convinced that toxic exposures from local subsistence fish diets presented a serious problem: "It wasn't like they needed convincing anymore. Now it was whether the data we collected was 'good enough' for them" (Swanston 2000). The EPA found the community data useable enough to generate a fish consumption rate for G/W residents in grams per day. The community survey data was found to be consistent with fish consumption rates from other urban areas where residents relied on subsistence diets of locally caught fish (Burger, Staine, and Gochfeld 1993; EPA 1999a, b).

The agency also gathered toxicological information on the fish species from New York State Department of Environmental Conservation (NYS DEC) studies, which estimated contaminant concentrations in East River fish (NYS DEC 1996). The EPA took fish samples from the East River and performed their own toxicological tests. Finally, contamination levels were estimated based on previous DEC measurements (NYS DEC 1996). Recognizing the fallibility of local knowledge, the EPA used these procedures to check the claims coming from residents. Thus, local knowledge altered the questions EPA professionals were asking and forced them to ask new questions about the data that were previously ignored.

Combining the local and professional data, EPA determined that the contaminants of concern in the locally caught fish included cadmium, mercury, chlordane, DDT, dieldrin, dioxins, PCBs, arsenic, and lead. However, arsenic was removed from the analysis since, according to

EPA, "much of the arsenic in edible fish is present as arsenic-containing organic compounds . . . and these organic forms of arsenic are generally not considered a threat to human health" (EPA 1999a). And, since lead exposures were slated to be analyzed in a separate, multiple-media study under the CEP, lead was also removed from the fish contaminant analysis (EPA 1999a).

Resident exposures then were calculated based on tissue contaminant concentrations found in the fish samples and based on the observed and calculated consumption rates. High- and low-end consumption rates for both adults and children were calculated in order to develop a range of exposure estimates. Combining the survey data with previous EPA studies, the agency derived exposure estimates for G/W anglers and their families. The calculations found that exposure to toxic contaminants for local anglers and their families exceeded EPA's oral reference doses (RfD), which generally serve as benchmark levels for noncancer health effects, for all contaminants except cadmium at both low- and high-end consumption estimates. Exposures to dioxins were particularly high. For example, the EPA reference dose for dioxin is 1×10^{-9} (mg/kg/day) while the estimated exposure level for the average high-end adult eating locally caught fish in G/W is 8.2×10^{-8} (mg/kg/day) and for the average high-end child fish consumer 1.5×10^{-7} (mg/kg/day) (EPA 1999a).

As part of CEP, the EPA decided to generate a lifetime cancer risk for local subsistence anglers. The lifetime cancer risk for adult subsistence anglers in G/W exceeded one in 10,000 (1×10^{-4}) for every exposure scenario. For subsistence anglers at the high-end consumption rate, the estimated individual lifetime cancer risk across all contaminants ranged from 8.7×10^{-2} for the single species maximum contaminant concentration to 5.8×10^{-3} for the minimum contaminant concentration. Using the cross-species average contaminant concentration, the estimated individual lifetime cancer risk for the high-end fish consumer (table 3.2) was 4.2×10^{-2}, and 6.0×10^{-3} for the low-end fish consumer (EPA 1999a).

Local Action with Local Knowledge

Without the community-generated information, the EPA likely would have overlooked this potentially serious health hazard. In their final

Table 3.2
Greenpoint/Williamsburg Angler Health Risks

Individual lifetime cancer risk	Low-end consumer	High-end consumer
Consumer of a single fish species	5.8×10^{-3}	8.7×10^{-2}
Consumer of multiple fish species	6.0×10^{-3}	4.2×10^{-2}

analysis, the EPA arrayed the results of the individual exposure assessments to show the range of contaminant exposures that exceeded health benchmark levels (EPA 1999a). While the results were compelling, the community group already had begun to act to prevent these exposures before the EPA analysis was complete.

While the EPA spent over five years completing the study in G/W, the Watchperson Project did not wait that long to take precautionary and preventative action. As their survey interview data began to suggest just how many residents were eating fish from the river, the Watchperson Project organized a series of "fish-in" days to educate anglers about potential toxic contamination in the fish they were eating (Waterfront Week 1999). Educational materials, printed in English and Spanish, described possible health risks from eating locally caught fish and suggested such things as cleaning and cooking techniques that might reduce contaminant intake (Swanston 2000). The Watchperson Project partnered on these efforts with the local chapter of the Sierra Club and other community environmental groups including Neighbors Against Garbage and the Friends of the India Street Pier. To ensure that the issue of subsistence fishing reached a larger audience, the Watchperson Project, working with the Sierra Club and NBC News, filmed a program on the health risks from subsistence fishing and swimming in the East River. This television program aired on Labor Day (Swanston 2000). In addition, the Watchperson Project began working with other groups in the area to identify alternative sources of food for subsistence anglers, such as community gardening.

The community group not only significantly altered and improved the EPA exposure assessment to take account of a hazard that would have been ignored, the effort also influenced EPA actions elsewhere. The community data, accounts from local anglers, and exposure assessment results have become a central piece of the EPA's and the NYS DEC's Hudson River Estuary Plan (EPA 1999a). The efforts also have changed the State DEC's approach to issuing and communicating fish advisories in the neighborhood and other communities along the Hudson River estuary. The work of the Watchperson Project has helped the State begin to develop a culturally sensitive fish-advisory program.

The community group's interviews of local subsistence angers revealed that the reasons they ate fish from the local river were complex; a combination of poverty, cultural tradition, and dietary habits all contributed to most anglers' accounts of why they ate potentially dangerous fish. Swanston understood that conventional fish advisories, which were already in existence before the EPA assessment, were not working in low-income, ethnic, urban neighborhoods such as G/W:

Telling anglers to just stop eating these fish, while maybe the safest thing, just isn't a reality for many of them. For some families the fish are their primary source of protein. Lots of fisherman were immigrants from the Caribbean and, being from the island of Nevis myself, I know fishing means more than just a meal. It is part of our identity. We've been working with the DEC to get them to integrate these understandings into their fish advisory programs. (Swanson 2000)

Changes in the EPA assessment and the DEC programs would not have occurred without information from local anglers gathered by the community organization.

The Cognitive Contribution of Community Knowledge

In this case, the resident's local knowledge successfully influenced (and improved) professional decision making (table 3.3). First, the community's involvement with the CEP reframed the original dietary exposure assessment and pushed the EPA to more closely reflect "lived reality." What seemed obvious to any community member, or even a visitor to the neighborhood— that the numerous distinct ethnic groups who lived in G/W made the neighborhood an extraordinary community—was missed by the EPA.

Residents convinced EPA that local culture contributed to a new exposure that the agency had not considered. Practice also changed when the Watchperson Project convinced the EPA that locals were capable of gathering appropriate information about anglers. Not only was local knowledge

Table 3.3
Cognitive Contribution of Community and Angler Knowledge: Selected Examples

---

1) Epistemology
Angler information extended the EPA risk assessment by including hazard data previously overlooked and debunking the assumption that lack of data equals lack of a hazard.
a) Aggregation
Local knowledge pointed out that the EPA's "urban default diet" was too general a level of aggregation for assessing dietary exposures.
b) Heterogeneity
Community members gathered angler data by age and ethnicity enabling the risk assessment to estimate hazards for different subpopulations.
c) Lifestyle
The EPA considered urban fishing a lifestyle issue, not a source of hazard data, and only changed its mind after community members took agency members on a tour of the neighborhood's piers.
d) Tacit knowledge
Angler information was from a hard-to-reach population that was reluctant to cooperate with outsiders because they feared deportation, did not speak English, and were embarrassed by the poverty-driven practice.
2) Procedural democracy
Community and angler voices that were previously excluded became an integral part of the assessment.
3) Effectiveness
The Watchperson Project performed educational campaigns, identified alternative food sources for angler families, and advised agencies on developing culturally sensitive fishing advisories.
4) Distributive justice
Community knowledge changed the risk assessment from one about estimating acceptable dietary risks to one focusing on which population groups were most at risk.

---

used to reframe the scope of the assessment, but it changed who was qualified to gather information. Locals became "equally expert" in assessing a practice within their own community.

The narratives behind local fishing practices convinced the EPA to develop a separate exposure assessment for subsistence anglers. Again, local knowledge influenced professional practice. Commonly, in risk assessment an absence of data leads to an assumption of an absence of harm; without any information about a hazard, the potential harm is, by default, ignored. In this case, the locally gathered data filled an information gap and an absence of data did not lead to an assumption of an absence of harm.

Finally, the results of the exposure assessment continue to influence the EPA, which funded a community waterfront-cleanup project sponsored by the Watchperson Project. The community group assisted the EPA and DEC in developing culturally sensitive fish advisories for the entire Hudson River Estuary. The EPA also has used information from the Watchperson Project interviews and surveys in a new guidance book aimed at educating local health departments about urban anglers (Swanston 2001).

Professional Uptake of Street Science

Why did the *street science* of community residents have an influence on professionals? The Watchperson Project organized concerned residents into a coalition that both raised the issue of subsistence fish diets and gathered angler data to back up their anecdotal evidence. Anglers also were organized for the first time, enabling the community group to document their practices. The knowledge local activists gathered consisted of both stories of anglers and statistical survey data. The narratives reflected what residents already knew and the quantitative data allowed the EPA to find a way of incorporating local narratives into the exposure assessment. Both types of information worked to fill gaps and allowed the study to more closely reflect how exposures are experienced by community members. The epistemological contribution is one of extending science; the community-sponsored data provided more accurate dietary information than the EPA was able to collect on its own. It produced an assessment of a hazard that would have been missed without local input.

The street science of local residents also was influential with professionals because it was linked to the larger environmental-justice movement. Activists in G/W characterized the initial CEP research methodology as insensitive to local culture. They claimed it was another example of government ignoring the plight of the poor and people of color, noting how the agency overlooked whether there might be local diets consisting primarily of locally caught fish. The activists were able to frame CEP as an environmental-justice issue by linking the local project

to ongoing debate over cumulative-risk assessment and exposure disparities nationwide. The Watchperson Project had gained credibility as an
environmental-justice organization with the EPA because the group had
been involved in the DEP's earlier environmental benefits program and in
a DOJ investigation into the fairness of siting a waste-transfer station in
the neighborhood.

Another factor that contributed to the success of locals was that the
Watchperson Project and its director acted as intermediary, translating
local experiences into terms that professional decision makers could take
seriously. The group brought the concerns of residents to the EPA and
volunteered to organize the angler survey. In particular, Samara
Swanston, the group's executive director, was someone who was able to
manage the organizing of local knowledge and its uptake into professional domains. As a lawyer with training in environmental health,
Swanston had legitimacy within both circles. She had been intimately
involved in the BAEL with the DEP, where she "cut her teeth" on community cumulative-hazard assessments. She also had gained the respect
of DEP staff through her involvement with the EBP, while retaining her
position as a strong community advocate by helping to organize a local
coalition to stop the siting of waste-transfer stations. As a woman of
color from the island of Nevis in the Caribbean, she had an intimate
knowledge of Caribbean-immigrant dietary and fishing practices. All
these factors contributed to her legitimacy with residents.

Finally, this effort was successful because the EPA had a relatively low-
cost way of responding to the challenges local knowledge presented to
their assessment. Adding the angler survey data to CEP did not require
the agency to radically alter its plans or even expend significant resources
collecting additional information. Moreover, the changes required low
or no political cost, since the agency already had announced that it was
committed to involving community members in a more meaningful way.
Further, the information locals offered was unlikely to assign blame for
any hazardous results on a particular industry or firm. The debate would
have been more politically charged if, for example, locals insisted on documenting discharges of waste into the river by local firms.

This chapter has highlighted how community residents organize local
knowledge into street science, borrowing from professional techniques,

exploring unquestioned assumptions, and ultimately extending science. Community members highlighted that only trusted local people would have access to honest information about angler practices and professionals recognized and valued the contribution of these street scientists. The next chapter explores the growing asthma epidemic in poor urban neighborhoods and how one community-based organized has tapped local knowledge to perform street science to better understand and manage the disease in a hard-hit Latino community.

4

Tapping Local Knowledge to Understand and Combat Asthma

When we said "health" they would ask us about some medical problem they were having. When they heard we were from El Puente, they would ask where they should send their kids for school next year or where they could get free food to feed their family that evening. We had to know where the food kitchens were, the drug-counselors, church leaders, you know? If we couldn't answer or at least send them to someone who could, they weren't going to trust us or talk to us. Before we even got to the questionnaire they wanted us to help them. Knowing how to do a survey about asthma was only part of what we did.
—Cecilia Iglesias Garden, Coordinator of El Puente's Community Health Educators, describing their community asthma survey in Williamsburg's Latino community

This chapter follows the work and street science of El Puente, a high-school and community-based organization in Williamsburg, to address the neighborhood's asthma epidemic. Combining community health surveys, focus-group meetings, folk medicinal practices and street art, El Puente members became street scientists investigating potential causes, triggers, and effective treatments for asthma. This chapter highlights the important role of community health workers in the street science process and how community knowledge can contribute to effective local action in the face of great scientific uncertainty.

Professional Health Assessments in Greenpoint/Williamsburg

The first environmental health studies in G/W came out of the community advisory committee meetings of the NYC Department of Environmental Protection's Environmental Benefits Program. The community advisors to the EBP, which included the Watchperson Project and El Puente, requested that the DEP sponsor a health study in the neighborhood. The representatives asked that the study look at cancer, lead poisoning, birth defects, and asthma, and in 1992 two studies reviewing available health data were conducted by the City University of New York (CUNY) Medical School in conjunction with the NYC Department of Health (DOH).

The health studies came in the wake of a protracted and contentious battle between the City and G/W community groups over the operation of an incinerator in the neighborhood (McFadden 1992).[24] With the incinerator battle still being waged in court, the study was released. It found few statistically elevated rates of asthma hospitalizations in the neighborhood (Kaminsky et al. 1993). Almost as soon as the health study was released, community activists challenged some of its findings, particularly the fact that the study of asthma hospitalizations only reviewed data from the local hospital, Woodhull Medical Center. According to locals, this was an institution that residents rarely visited for medical treatment. Indeed, residents noted that Woodhull had a "bad reputation" and a study that relied only on asthma hospitalizations from this institution could not accurately characterize what was happening in the neighborhood.

In the same year the DOH/CUNY health studies were released, El Puente started a high school called the Academy for Peace and Social Justice. The high school's curriculum was geared toward learning and action for social change, and community health and environmental justice became one focal point of the high school's curriculum. Students created an environmental group called the Toxic Avengers. Science classes were spent studying a neighborhood facility that stored radioactive waste and the health effects of air pollution. Students helped organize a protest on the Williamsburg Bridge to raise awareness about a proposed incinerator. They also tracked daily air-quality measurements from a monitoring station on the roof of their building.

Science students at El Puente were interested in trying to draw a connection between local air pollution and community health problems, particularly asthma. Nearly every student either had asthma or had a family member with the disease (Penchaszadeh 1999). In order to try and make the pollution-health connection, El Puente knew it would need help. For assistance they turned to a nonprofit group that specialized in helping communities perform epidemiological studies, called Community Information and Epidemiological Technologies (CIET). El Puente chose CIET, according to John Fleming, former program director at El Puente, because they had worked for two decades performing community-health research in Mexico, their staff spoke Spanish, and they understood Latin culture. Additionally, one of their principal investigators, Robert Ledogar, was based in New York City and was interested in partnering with a Latino community in the United States. El Puente and CIET set out to explore the relationships between local air pollution and public health and to reveal the weaknesses in the DOH/CUNY health study.

El Puente and CIET received funding from the Nathan Cummings Foundation to develop a general health survey for high school students to perform among their peers, family, and El Puente members. This survey did not mention the word asthma, but an overwhelming number of responses identified asthma as their top health concern. El Puente and CIET recognized that to make any connections between asthma and air pollution, they needed to survey the entire community and have the assistance of more than just students and volunteers.

After El Puente's first survey was complete and while they were planning a follow-up survey, the NYC DOH launched the New York City Childhood Asthma Initiative. The Asthma Initiative was the result of pressure from physicians and community groups contending that the City had no coordinated program to address what appeared to be a growing asthma epidemic afflicting many of NYC's school children (O'Neill 1996). The City program was also a response to a *New York Daily News* investigative report, which revealed that most City public schools lacked nurses trained in treating asthmatic students and the schools had no asthma-education program, despite asthma being the leading cause of school absenteeism (Calderone et al. 1998; Carr 1992; De Palo 1994). El Puente was eligible for a grant from the Asthma Initiative, and the community group used this support to organize a community-wide asthma survey.

In order to explore the possibility of a community-wide survey investigating asthma rates, El Puente organized a meeting of the Community Alliance for the Environment (CAFE). This coalition consisted of a number of community organizations in G/W and originally came together in the early 1990s to stop a proposed incinerator. The coalition brought together the neighborhood's different cultural and ethnic groups and their representative organizations: The Polish and Slavic Center, representing those immigrants; United Jewish Organization, representing the Hasidic Jewish community; and El Puente, representing Latinos. When El Puente suggested a community-wide survey, the other groups balked, each for different cultural reasons. The Hasidim were reluctant to talk publicly about health issues, and the Poles and Slavs were not comfortable with having strangers interview them in their homes. While CAFE failed to reach agreement on one community-wide asthma project, each group decided to do something on their own.

El Puente developed a community-asthma survey targeting the Latino population in Williamsburg's Southside and used the survey as a community-organizing tool. Since considerable disagreement persists over the causes of asthma, designing a survey was challenging for El Puente. The next section briefly reviews the debates over asthma in the medical community to provide some context to the choices El Puente made in their own research.

The Epidemiology of Asthma

For immunologists, epidemiologists, and others in public health professions, asthma has become a fascinating mystery (Pearce et al. 1998; Shell 2000). At a time when biomedicine claims to have a handle on controlling the spread of infectious disease, chronic diseases like asthma remain unstoppable (Hegner 2000). Asthma is the most common chronic childhood disease in the developed world, affecting approximately 10 million children under 16 years old in the United States (Woolcock and Peat 1997). Between 1982 and 1992, the prevalence rate for pediatric asthma (under 18 years of age) in the United States increased by 58%. The mortality rate from asthma for persons 19 years of age and under increased by 78% from 1980 to 1993 (IOM 2000). Although asthma was the tenth most common principal diagnosis in emergency department visits among all patients in 1996, asthma led in emergency-department visits for children, excluding accidents (Noble 1999).

Asthma is particularly prevalent in urban and racial/ethnic minority populations (Miller et al. 2000). In the United States, the asthma hospitalization and morbidity rates for nonwhites are more than twice those for whites. The activity limitation rate due to asthma is 30% higher in African Americans than any other group (Eggleston et al. 1999). The causes of increased morbidity and the differential risk for urban, racial/ethnic minority populations are not well understood.

New York City has one of the highest rates of asthma in the United States. Rates are especially high among Latino and African-American children, and asthma has become the leading cause of hospital admissions for NYC school-aged children (NYC DOH 2003). A Mount Sinai Medical Center study examined NYC rates of hospital admission for asthma by ethnicity (Crain et al. 1994). Asthma admission rates were found to have increased by 12.7% in 3 years, and mortality had also increased. Asthma hospitalization rates were 7.5 times higher for minorities than for whites. This same study found that the Bronx and Upper Manhattan (Harlem) had the highest asthma admission rates in all of the city, with East Harlem and Williamsburg second and third, respectively (Claudio et al. 1999).

In Central Harlem, the problem is particularly acute. Recent work by Columbia University and the Harlem Children's Zone, a community-based organization, found that nearly 1 in 4 children had asthma. After screening and surveying 1,982 children aged 0–12 in 2003, the Harlem Children's Zone Asthma Initiative found that over 28% of these children had been told by a doctor or nurse that they had asthma, and 30% had asthma and/or asthma-like symptoms, 24% had missed school due to asthma in the last 14 days, and nearly 35% had visited the emergency room in the last 3 months for treatment of asthma (Nicolas et al. 2003).

While debate continues over whether the rise in asthma rates is due to a change in reporting or increased awareness by patients and physicians, definitions of the disease remain elusive. Asthma remains a particularly difficult disease because its principal causes are difficult to isolate (Pearce et al. 1998). The Institute of Medicine describes asthma as a chronic disease characterized by inflammation of the airways and lungs that causes attacks of wheezing and shortness of breath (IOM 2000). However, no scientific consensus exists over what *causes* asthma development. Allergens, irritants, environmental tobacco smoke, air pollution, and a host of other factors are suspected "triggers" that increase the severity of the disease, but no single or constellation of these triggers has been identified as the leading cause. With so little known about asthma, scientists are often uncertain about whether asthma is one or a number of different diseases that have a common clinical picture—the set of symptoms or characteristics physicians use to make a diagnosis (NIH 2003).

One dominant hypothesis takes a biomedical approach to the disease and claims that compared to non-asthmatics, asthmatics are more atopic—having a genetically determined hypersensitivity to environmental allegens—and that allergens are the primary trigger and likely cause of the disease.[25] This theory states that the immune system "overreacts" to certain allergens, producing chemicals such as leukotrienes, which cause inflammation in the airways of the lungs, narrowing of airways, and excessive mucus production (Pearce et al. 1998). Cockroach allergens found in household dust, along with dust mites, cats, and pollens (e.g., ragweed and rye grass) are suspected to be the leading allergens that both cause and trigger childhood asthma morbidity and mortality (Gergen and Weiss 1995). The proponents of this theory also claim that these particular allergens are more likely to be found in the dirty, dilapidated homes of poor, inner-city children, explaining the distribution of the disease among these populations (Platts-Mills 1999). Yet, another take on the cause of asthma from a biomedical viewpoint argues that early childhood exposure to allergens helps *prevent* the onset of asthma by building immunities, and that the parents of poor, inner-city children are not exposing them *enough* to allergens at an early age (Rosenstreich et al. 1997). However, neither explanation suggests why different asthma rates appear *among* African-Americans and Latino populations in the United States (Pearce et al. 2000).

A second hypothesis, often called the behavioral or lifestyle framework, claims that asthma occurrence is the result of an individual choice about a way of living (Rosenstreich et al. 1997). A leading lifestyle theory for explaining asthma distribution claims that societal excess has led people to not exercise, to eat a poor diet of fatty foods and, because they are inside more often, to increase their exposure to harmful allergens such as environmental tobacco smoke and dust mites. This hypothesis suggests that the children of America's worst—off groups—such as those in poverty and people of color—are most likely to spend time indoors, and the more children stay inside, the higher their exposure to the triggers of asthma, such as indoor allergens, tobacco smoke, gas from open pilot lights, and chemicals from cleaning solvents (Platts-Mills 1999).

A third set of hypotheses claim that the causes of asthma rest in the "environment" (Eggleston et al. 1999). One environmental theory suggests that dirty indoor air, including allergens and environmental tobacco smoke, is the leading cause of asthma. This hypothesis states that in the homes of the urban poor, common overcrowding contributes to dirt, dust, mold, humidity, and mildew, all of which instigate harmful allergens (Gergen et al. 1999). Combustion effluents from residential gas stoves, especially oxides of nitrogen (NO_2) also are blamed for respiratory symptoms and reduced lung function in populations of both healthy and asthmatic children (Delfino 2002). Yet, another contradictory "environmental" hypothesis states that *excessive* indoor hygiene is the leading cause of asthma. In this view, modern hygienic practices such as industrial cleaning agents and solvents have eliminated the "useful" microbes and parasites that challenge but ultimately strengthen the human immune system and, absent these useful microbes, children are less protected from developing asthma (Carpenter 1999).

Other explanations that fall under the banner of "environment" claim that outdoor air pollution is a leading cause of asthma (Leikauf 2002). Low-level ozone causes airway inflammation and hyperactivity, bronchial epithelial permeability, decrements in pulmonary function, cough, chest tightness, pain on inspiration, and upper-respiratory-tract irritation (ATS 1996; Vedal et al. 1998). Epidemiologic studies undertaken in a variety of locations indicate a relationship between outdoor air pollution and adverse respiratory effects in children, including asthma. The pollutants most frequently implicated in these studies have been respirable particles, ozone, and hazardous air pollutants (Holgate et al. 1999).

An analysis of the U.S. EPA's nonattainment regions for national ambient-air-quality standards found that Latinos and African Americans are more likely than whites to live in areas that exceed federal standards for many toxic pollutants such as lead, ozone, carbon monoxide, and particulates (Wernette and Nieves 1992). The disparities that these authors found are significant. For example, the percentage of the population that live in areas of nonattainment for ozone is 52% for whites, 62% for African Americans, and 71% for Latinos. The pattern is similar for a variety of other air pollutants. This finding is important for understanding children's environmental health, as levels of ambient-air pollution, such as particulate matter and ozone, have been shown to correlate with morbidity from respiratory illness (Ostro et al. 2001). One hypothesis claims that while overall quality of ambient air has improved, an uneven distribution of localized air pollutants persists, and this may explain some of the increased rates of respiratory disease found especially among minority and poor children (IOM 2000). A study by the American Lung Association found that 61% of pediatric asthma cases occur in children who live in areas of nonattainment for air-quality standards as defined by the U.S. EPA (ALA 1993).

Clearly, asthma is a disease that remains highly uncertain in the scientific and policy communities. David Satcher, the Surgeon General, noted in 1999:

One of the real issues is, why are we seeing this increase in asthma? And we don't know the answer to that. Until you understand why you have an increase, and you have documented it, it is very hard to say you have a strategy that is going to make a difference.[26]

Understanding asthma rates and triggers in the Greenpoint/ Williamsburg neighborhood has proved equally challenging.

Professional Analyses of Neighborhood Asthma

The asthma study in G/W performed by the NYC DOH and the CUNY Medical School's Department of Community Health and Social Medicine was intended to determine the prevalence of neighborhood asthma. The study calculated the percentage of residents in all census tracts in G/W who visited Woodhull Medical Center at least once for asthma between 1987 and 1991 (Kaminsky et al. 1992, 1993). The study revealed that the percentage of the population in any census tract in G/W who visited Woodhull for asthma in the years 1987 to 1992 never exceeded 4.35% (Kaminsky et al. 1993, 13). The report also notes that the census tracts in G/W with the highest percentage of the population visiting Woodhull for

asthma were tracts 487 and 507, with 89% and 97% Latino populations, respectively (Kaminsky et al. 1993, 13, 75). Of the five census
tracts with the highest percentage of asthma visits to Woodhull, all were
over 75% Latino, with an average Latino population of 86% (Kaminsky
et al. 1993, 13, 47). The report also notes that these same five census
tracts had the lowest median family income of all the tracts in G/W.
While the report noted that these findings were not statistically significant and there did not appear to be an asthma problem in the neighborhood, the report did include the caveat that "not all persons with asthma
go to Woodhull for treatment" and "while these data provide an accurate picture of where Woodhull asthma patients live, they do not reflect
the total number of persons with asthma in Greenpoint/Williamsburg"
(Kaminsky et al. 1993, 18).

For many at El Puente and others in the community who eagerly anticipated the results of this study, the "caveat" of the asthma findings
seemed to be more of a "gross inaccuracy." From the outset community
members dismissed the study for failing to aggregate results by age,
gender, and ethnicity and, perhaps most importantly, for only using hospitalization data from a local hospital which "most neighborhood residents rarely if ever visit" (Penchaszadeh 2001). Among longstanding
Latinos and Hasidic Jews in the neighborhood, that Woodhull was a hospital to be avoided was common knowledge. According to one long time
resident:

For as long as I've lived in this community, we've [Dominican population] avoided
Woodhull. It was just a scary place. I mean we used to joke as kids that if you were
bad they were going to send you there. Nobody I know ever goes to Woodhull.

Community-health-survey findings that El Puente would later publish
supported these stories; the survey found that over 75% of Southside
Latino residents reported visiting a hospital for asthma outside the community, not Woodhull. In Kranzler's (1995, 68) history of Hasidic
Williamsburg, he notes that Woodhull was the only center treating men-
tally ill Hasidim, but was avoided by Hasidim for almost all other health
problems.

By ignoring this local knowledge the DOH study couldn't offer a por-
trayal of asthma treatment that reflected local practice. The study seemed
to undermine, rather than enhance, neighborhood trust in the agencies

and experts who were supposed to protect them. Wynne (1996, 51) has noted that studies intended to placate weary publics often do just the opposite: "Institutions which can be seen to be reconstructing history so as to confirm their own blamelessness whilst attempting to manufacture public trust and legitimation are prima facie likely to be undermining public trust rather than enhancing it." The DOH/CUNY asthma study seemed to further alienate residents from professional decision makers and contributed to locals taking their own action to understand the disease.

El Puente's Community-Health-Survey Philosophy

Community members were disappointed that the professional health studies did not align with their experiences with asthma nor provide a possible explanation for why the disease seemed to be increasing at alarming rates for most local children. The studies, like most traditional epidemiological study designs, searched for individual causes of cases, as opposed to population distributions of incidence. This research approach tends to ignore how extra-individual contextual factors, such as neighborhood pollution, housing conditions, violence, and deteriorating infrastructure might contribute to disease above and beyond individual characteristics or lifestyles (Diez Roux 1998). When public-health researchers ignore these contextual characteristics, often referred to as ecological factors, explanations for distributions of disease tend to revolve around stories of individual responsibility and personal blame. In communities like G/W experiencing disproportionate environmental-hazard and disease burdens, one result is that already disenfranchised populations feel further alienated from science and the institutions supporting technical solutions to environmental health problems. Omar Freilla, an environmental-justice activist in the South Bronx, described the political impact of professional studies that ignore local realities:

On the one hand you have a lot of researchers following their own questions, legitimate questions that need to be answered. The problem is when you have a good question being asked, but the people who are responsible for implementing some sort of solution purposely put it in a context where they don't have to do anything. Government agencies don't want to look at asthma as an air pollution problem because then they'd have to do something about it. (quoted from McGowan 1999)

A similar sentiment, which emerged in Williamsburg after the release of the academic studies, acted as a key impetus behind El Puente's community-health-survey project (Fleming 1999).

El Puente's survey approach aimed to empower individuals to investigate the local factors that might be contributing to asthma while emphasizing specific actions that residents and the community-based organization could take to mitigate the impact of the disease (Ledogar 2001). According to Luis Garden-Acosta, executive director of El Puente, their health research "stems from the conviction that science should be used as an instrument for collective self-help" (Ledogar, Garden-Acosta, and Penchaszadeh 1999, 1795). The asthma research was also an extension of the organization's ongoing environmental-health and-justice program, which included such issues as stopping neighborhood waste-transfer stations, cleaning up derelict brownfield sites and creating community gardens (Fleming 2000).

El Puente and CIET adopted a research methodology called Sentinel Community Surveys or Service Delivery Surveys (Freire 1974; Ledogar and Andersson 1993). In these methods a mix of quantitative and qualitative data is gathered by existing community organizations, which are trained to conduct questionnaires, face-to-face interviews, and public discussions of survey design and results—all with the intention of collective action (Fals Borda and Rahman 1991). According to CIET, the methodology includes:

data collection cycles to be repeated at regular intervals. Local researchers become increasingly capable of conducting these surveys themselves. With each new cycle, information on the previous cycle is disseminated to communities. Over time, success of solutions derived from previous cycles can be measured, and topics for investigation gradually broadened. In this way, the methodology provides the basis for sustained, critical dialogue on issues that affect people's daily lives. (CIET 2000)

The research philosophy is rooted in the Latin American tradition of participatory action research (PAR), which emphasizes that research ought to be understood as a process of education and pedagogy should be a practice of social transformation (Freire 1974; Fals Borda and Rahman 1991). The techniques used in PAR include listening, observation, community meetings, socio-dramas, critical recovery of history, valuing and applying folk culture, and the production and diffusion of new knowledge through written, oral, and visual forms (Chambers 1997, 108). El Puente adopted an aspect of PAR called "listening research." In this technique, teams of community residents, trained by research scientists, combine their training with their own skills in observation, questioning, semistructured interviewing, and group discussions in order to gather data (Ledogar 1999). The group also used a technique from Freire (1974) called "thematic investigation," where local data are gathered by community residents and the information is then discussed in groups settings. In these dialogues, the gathered information is analyzed by community members for its local relevance and its relation to the larger community. This process continues in an iterative fashion until the community-gathered information is being examined in relation to local, state, and world affairs (Freire 1974, 80). According to Analia Penchaszadeh, director of environmental health programs at El Puente:

Fundamentally for us, what is important is to change relationships between community members and the powerful influence of expert science. Models that put the expert at the center of decision making, with all the power to define problems, result in actions dependent on the expert; either that or individuals are told what to do to solve their own problems. In our model, we seek to place power for conducting research and taking action within the group—the collective—not with an expert or only individuals. (Penchaszadeh 2000)

Between 1995 and 2000, El Puente conducted four surveys, with each building on the previous by incorporating community learning to develop new and more focused questions (Ledogar et al. 2000). The group limited their surveys to the Southside of Williamsburg, an approximately two-square-mile section of the five-square-mile G/W neighborhood in which a majority of the Latino population El Puente served lived. The Southside study area is bordered on the west by the East River, on the north by Metropolitan Avenue; on the east by Union Avenue, and on the south by Division Avenue (see figure I.1). In this corridor of Williamsburg, close to 85% of the population is Latino, a majority are of Dominican and Puerto Rican ancestry, and nearly 90% of the residents living in the Southside do not speak English as their primary language (Sexton 1998). Only 5% of Southside residents hold college degrees, and over half were receiving public assistance in 1997 (Sexton 1998). El Puente began its survey work in the Southside community it served, and the surveys were administered by those living in that community (Ledogar 1999).

In an effort to help students think about ways to make the connections between air pollution and public health, El Puente and CIET together developed a survey instrument. The CIET staff provided one based on their experience in developing countries, and the students and staff helped make it relevant to Williamsburg by providing information about what some of the constraints might be for soliciting information and who else in the community could help administer the survey and participate in follow-up discussions (Penchaszadeh 2000). Eventually, students, El Puente Academy faculty, and CIET developed a 28-item questionnaire focused on soliciting perceptions of community health.[27]

With financial assistance from the Nathan Cummings Foundation, 50 high-school students at El Puente Academy, five teachers, and five El Puente staff members performed door-to-door interviewing, reaching 280 households and 1,065 individuals in December of 1995 (El Puente-CIET 1995). The survey was performed in homes using face-to-face interviewing. A student teamed up with an adult to interview the respondent, normally the head of the household. Often the adults did not speak English, so the students helped in translation. All the data were statistically analyzed using the epidemiological software package *Epi Info*.

The survey revealed that residents felt that there were serious problems of air pollution and respiratory disease in the neighborhood, but most residents had not taken action, nor were they aware of any specific actions they could take, to address these conditions (table 4.1). For El Puente, community perceptions about pollution and the lack of information about available health-promoting activities suggested to the organization that a series of follow-up surveys were necessary to obtain more detailed information and to provide relevant health-promoting options for residents (Ledogar 2001). El Puente also recognized that surveying only the Southside population might not allow them to draw any conclusions about possible relationships between neighborhood environmental quality and public health. In order to do this, El Puente would need to expand the survey project to the entire G/W community.

Table 4.1
Select Survey Results, 1995 El Puente Household Survey

Survey question	Percentage of all respondents
Causes of pollution	
Vehicles	42%
Factories	17%
Garbage	10%
Solutions to pollution	
Recycling	40%
Reducing traffic	21%
Limiting factories	4%
Believe there is a serious air-quality problem	84%
Believe pollution in the neighborhood is heavy	60%
Smoker in household > 15 yrs	20%
Smokes inside	77%
Asthma sufferer in house	**26%**
Self-reported respiratory problem	18%
Self-reported asthma	13%
Think there is an air quality problem (of those with asthma)	70%

Attempting a Neighborhoodwide Asthma Survey

Soon after the completion of El Puente's first survey, the NYC DOH established its Childhood Asthma Initiative. The Initiative focused on educating community organizations and school children about asthma triggers and how to manage the disease (DOH 2000). The Initiative's mantra was: "I have asthma but asthma doesn't have me." Through this program, El Puente applied for and received financial support under the guise of asthma education. The monies were not intended to support a community-health survey, and according to Louise Cohen, director of the Initiative:

We were reluctant to support a community survey performed by a community organization because we felt they were just going to be disappointed after putting a lot of hard work into such a large undertaking. We felt the resources would be better spent on education and improving case management. El Puente insisted on a survey project and we compromised by agreeing that the survey should include the entire community. We figured a survey might be a good way to involve all the groups in Williamsburg in the Asthma Initiative. (Cohen 2000)

El Puente called a meeting of the Community Alliance for the Environment, a coalition of Latinos, Hasidic Jews, and Polish immigrants (Greider 1993). These three ethnic groups make up over 85% of the G/W population, but they live largely segregated from one another; the Latinos occupy the Southside, the Poles are in Greenpoint and the Northside, and the Hasidim occupy the Southside around the Navy Yard and East Williamsburg. At the CAFE meeting, the three community-based organizations representing each ethnic group were present: El Puente for the Latinos, United Jewish Appeal (UJO) for the Hasidic Jews, and the Polish-Slavic Center (PSC) for the Poles. Since each of these groups has a different mission, El Puente suspected that a collaborative asthma-research project might be met with some skepticism (Penchaszadeh 2001). For example, the PSC and UJO are community-service-provider organizations, which often implement city-funded programs for their constituent populations. El Puente, as a member organization, differs from these groups because the organization is also a community-learning center and home to a charter high school, but it is not a social service agency.

Almost from the outset, according to Rabbi David Niederman, executive director of UJO, the idea of a community-wide survey was problematic. The rabbi explained that the Satmar Hasidim lead a life largely isolated from the "outside" world, issues of health are not talked about publicly, and residents would be unlikely to open their doors to surveyors—even if they were Hasidim (Niederman 2001). He also explained that since most Hasidim are not educated in the sciences or human health, most would not possess the knowledge or language to describe asthma. Even more troubling, talking about a "disease" might immediately raise fears of death and create community panic. Niederman later described his opposition to the community survey to me:

Remember, we are not the Amish but really only one step away. What I mean is that we are a very insular community, more than any other of the Hasidim. There are no English newspapers, no TV, no Internet, no radios, no newstands. We have one Yiddish newspaper, and that is all people read. English is a second language for everyone. Most people have very little or even no exposure to the outside world. It is just not encouraged or valued here. So, talking about disease such as asthma is something that they are not familiar with or even comfortable talking about. When most hear disease it means "near-death" and public conversations about disease are just not part of our lives.

In our community we are very interdependent, and there is a fear of being stigmatized. God forbid you are known as the family with disease! This is a close-knit community and people are afraid of sharing certain information. When it comes to illness, unfortunately, we generally don't talk about it.[28]

The rabbi's statement highlights that accurate health information not only is deeply tied to group lifestyles, but may be unavailable to outsiders due to barriers such as language, customs, and trust. Instead of a survey, UJO advocated for an asthma-education program in the schools. This, it turned out, was something only they could provide because the schools for Hasidim are all privately run religious schools called Yeshivas where lessons are taught primarily in Yiddish and Hebrew.

Like UJO, the PSC was reluctant to engage in a community survey. Part of the problem for the PSC appeared to be ownership. Since El Puente was spearheading the project and already had CIET as a consultant, the PSC was concerned that the survey would reflect the values of El Puente and that the PSC might not have the chance to make the project sensitive to its community. In addition, according to Renata Jablonski, PSC asthma program director, the PSC was more interested in taking action against local truck traffic, waste-transfer stations, and sewage-treatment plants, all of which they believed were the principal causes of local health problems (Jablonski 1999). Eventually, the idea of a community-wide survey spearheaded by El Puente died when the other community organizations realized they could receive funding to do their own projects from the recently created NYC Childhood Asthma Initiative.

El Puente's Participatory Action-Research

After their 1995 survey and with the rejection of the idea of a community-wide survey, El Puente decided to hire a dedicated survey staff from the neighborhood in order to make the survey project a full-time community organizing and research endeavor (Ledogar et al. 1998). El Puente recruited community members to act as "health promoters" to administer the surveys, lead community discussions over interpretations of results, and help residents manage their asthma and health more generally. El Puente's objective was to hire community residents with long-standing ties, commitments, and knowledge of the neighborhood, including people who knew about available neighborhood social services. According to Cecilia Iglesias-Garden, former coordinator of El Puente's Community Health Educator (CHE) team, it was important that the health workers could speak credibly about more issues than just asthma:

We learned in the first survey that the first thing most people asked us when we came to their door had nothing to do with asthma. When we said "health" they would ask us about some medical problem they were having. When they heard we were from El Puente, they would ask where they should send their kids for school next year or where they could get free food to feed their family that evening. We had to know where the food kitchens were, the drug-counselors, church leaders, you know? If we couldn't answer or at least send them to someone who could, they weren't going to trust us or talk to us. Before we even got to the questionnaire they wanted us to help them. Knowing how to do a survey about asthma was only part of what we did. (Iglesias-Garden 2000)

Since the survey administrators needed to have an intimate "local knowledge" of the neighborhood and an interest in asthma, El Puente also looked to recruit community members with a personal or familial stake in asthma and those who "had a passion for improving the health of the community" (Iglesias-Garden 2001). Eventually, El Puente chose ten women from the community, all Spanish-speaking Puerto Ricans and Dominicans, to be part of the CHE team.

The CHE women were trained by CIET, the NYC DOH, and public-health professionals from Hunter College in the etiology of asthma, epidemiological methods, and how to facilitate community meetings about health. Since CIET and El Puente were committed to involving the CHE in survey design, administration, and analysis, the women also were trained in survey methods. The CHE team acted as community-health workers, not just survey administrators. Community-health workers, or *promotoras de salud,* are lay health advocates and advisors who learn from and help educate individuals and groups toward increased well-being (Frankel 1992; Witmer et al. 1995). They often combine personal life experiences managing illness with experiences of other community members to inform their work (Ramirez-Valles 1998). The workers act as bridge-builders between residents, cultural and folk practices, and professional providers of clinical health care and medication regimes (Love and Gardner 1997;

Farmer 1999). This can be accomplished when the CHE offer basic disease education, screening and detection techniques, translate the cultural and folk practices for health care providers unfamiliar with them, and seek professional health care for those who desire it. They can also improve the quality of care for those who often are intimidated by physicians by facilitating better communication between patients and health-care providers. In NYC Latino communities, the community-health-worker tradition dates to the Young Lords' "barefoot doctors" of the 1960s, who worked to raise public consciousness of lead poisoning in East Harlem (Melendez 2003). Community-health-worker models increasingly are being used for action research to address urban asthma (Hill, Bone, and Butz 1996; Parker et al. 2003; Nicolas et al. 2003).

With the CHE in place, El Puente performed a second survey, reaching 727 households and 2,311 individuals (Ledogar et al. 1998). The survey gathered both qualitative and quantitative information about local asthma that had never before been organized, and the quantitative data were again statistically analyzed using *Epi Info*. The survey found a 12.4% active-asthma rate for all Latinos living in the Southside, more than twice the national rate of 5.4% (Ledogar et al. 1999; Eggelston et al. 1999).[29] Other survey findings revealed that nearly 20% of women between the ages of 45 and 64 had been told by a doctor that they had asthma, 40% of asthma sufferers had gone to a hospital emergency room because of the disease in the 12 months prior to the survey, and 27% of these respondents visited the ER more than once (figure 4.1, table 4.2).

The survey also highlighted that asthma medication was taken often or daily by 41% of the population responding to the survey. Twenty percent of adults with asthma thought that something at their job was causing their breathing problems. Individuals over 14 years old who had lived in the neighborhood for 15 years or more were twice as likely to have asthma as those who had lived in Brooklyn for a shorter time. And, community residents who had moved to the neighborhood from the Dominican Republic, Puerto Rico, or other areas in Latin American, regardless of how recently, were only half as likely to have asthma as those who had moved to the neighborhood from within the continental United States. Yet, it was during focus-group discussions following the

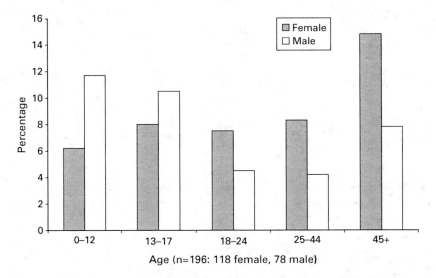

Figure 4.1.
Rates of active asthma by gender and age, 1998 El Puente Survey. Source: Ledogar, Garden-Acosta, and Penchaszadeh 1999.

surveys that El Puente began to uncover some of the specific local knowledge that provided the meanings, interpretations, and explanations behind the survey findings.

Focus Groups and the Mobilization of Local Knowledge

Focus groups were an integral part of El Puente's participatory information-gathering and data-analysis process. After each survey, a series of meetings were held where residents, the CHE team, and CIET discussed specific survey findings. The topics of the meetings were chosen by the CHE team and focused on survey findings or interesting information that the surveyors heard in the community (Ledogar 2000). The idea behind these community dialogues was that "the survey process was incomplete without community members helping to give life to the numbers as analysts and without local people learning about the findings and, most importantly, helping strategize over what to do about these problems" (Penchaszadeh 2001). Each focus-group meeting was an

Table 4.2
Comparison of Selected Results from El Puente Community Surveys

Survey question	1995	1998	1999	1999 national means
People	1,065	2,311	3,015	
Households	280	727	946	
Told by MD in last 12 months that have asthma (all ages/sex)[a]	N/A	8.4%	8.3%	
Do not have health insurance	N/A	N/A	45%	
Rely on Medicaid	N/A	67%	73%	
Self-reported asthma (all ages/sex)	N/A	12.4%	11.9%	5.4%
0–4 (n=280)	N/A	11.1%	14.4%	5.8%
5–14 (n=672)	N/A	14.1%	15.3%	7.4%
15–34 (n=1011)	N/A	12.4%	9.3%	5.2%
35–64 (n=875)	N/A	13%	12.3%	4.5%
65+ (n=165)	N/A	15.8%	11.9%	4.5%
Take asthma meds daily or often	N/A	41%	44%	
Use home remedies	N/A	N/A	43%	
Use home remedies and take asthma prescription medications		N/A	90%	
Do not discuss home-remedy use with MD		N/A	67%	

a. Defined as active asthma, which includes: one or more asthma symptoms (wheezing, sleep disturbance, speaking difficulty) in the past 12 months; taking asthma medication frequently or every day; having been to the emergency room for asthma in past 12 months

informal community dialogue run by the CHE team where the young and old, asthma sufferers and those without the disease, came together to work on the problem collectively.

El Puente's objective was to create a forum where residents were in control of the subject matter and the dialogue. The forums were intentionally designed to address the loss of control over pollution and health issues that El Puente learned about in their first survey by emphasizing actions individuals could take to address the disease. According to Iglesias-Garden:

The discussions were about the survey but also about people gaining control of their own well-being. You know, many poor Latinos feel their health is out of their control. Getting control of your own health, or at least talking about it, was a real act of resistance and empowerment. The focus groups were about discussing survey information as much as about sharing stories of what people could do. Yeah, the focus groups were about the asthma survey, but more so they were about challenging complacency and sharing stories of ownership over your health. (Iglesias-Garden 2000)

In order to encourage discussions of resistance and ownership, the CHE team focused on soliciting information that only local people could provide. For example, one survey finding was that women over 45 years old had a high prevalence of asthma, similar to that found in children. This was surprising since children, not middle-aged women, are generally suspected as being the most vulnerable to developing asthma. During discussions El Puente learned that the only work usually available to these women was in laundries, dry cleaners, beauty salons, or "sweatshop" textile factories—all occupations with potentially dangerous air pollutants. These occupational environments typically expose workers to solvents, heat, humidity, and dust that all have proved to contribute to respiratory illnesses. Many women revealed in the discussions that they took these jobs because of their immigrant status, language barriers, or because "that was where women in the community could easily find work."

The group discussions turned to what El Puente and the affected women might do to avoid these exposures, and included everything from learning about health and safety standards, unionizing, challenging typical gender roles and assumptions, and learning a new "marketable" skill (Iglesias-Garden 2001). The women also talked about what additional information El Puente might want to collect in subsequent surveys and focus groups to learn more about why women over 45 had elevated rates of asthma. In many cases, the focus groups allowed previously passive women to speak out and share stories about their employment dilemmas, illness, and feelings of disempowerment more generally (Penchaszadeh 2001). Without the focus-group discussions, it is unlikely that the potential relationships between women's occupations and asthma would have been revealed or that there would have been an opportunity for the silent suffering of local women to be shared.

Latino Home Remedies

El Puente's third survey reached 3,015 people in 946 households. The survey gathered more detailed demographic information about the Southside and found that 47% of the households identified themselves as Dominican, 42% Puerto Rican, 6% other Latino, and less than 5% Other (table 4.3). The survey also revealed that 30% of people did not have any health insurance; nearly 50% of all children in Mexican, Central American, and South American families, and 40% of Dominican children were not insured. Overall, the survey found that 19% of all children 19 years of age or younger were uninsured. In addition, over 66% of respondents reported using herbal or some other home remedy to treat their asthma. Whether insured or not, over 56% of Dominicans and 45% of Puerto Ricans had substituted a home remedy for physician-prescribed medication. The widespread use of home remedies and why residents were replacing prescribed medication with traditional home remedies became the topic of the next series of follow-up focus-group discussions.

El Puente chose to emphasize home-remedies in their survey and during group discussions because it was an issue that almost all community members had knowledge of and, according to one CHE team member, "almost everyone [CHE members] felt like they could speak credibly about home-remedies because they had experience with them." Practitioners of herbal medicine from Puerto Rico, the Dominican Republic, Ecuador, and other Central American countries were invited to the meetings. For many of the practitioners it was the first time they had been asked to share their knowledge in public. Importantly, the focus-group process allowed those often marginalized in community-health decision-making, particularly women folk healers, to become valued participants in the research process. According to one woman:

I've been using these remedies for as long as I can remember. My grandmother told me what to do and I tell the children. It was all passed down by word of mouth. Like a recipe. You remember what works; maybe add a little more or less here or there, but that was it. If you were from a certain region in Puerto Rico, everyone used the same treatments, so it was taken for granted that your neighbor knew what you were doing or talking about.

Table 4.3
Selected Results from 1999 El Puente Survey

	Dominican and other Latino		Puerto Rican	
	Asthma	No asthma	Asthma	No asthma
Asthma period prevalence	5.3%		13.2%	
Age group by sex				
0–12				
Female	9.7%	14.8%	15%	12%
Male	26.9%	13.5%	17%	12.6%
13–24				
Female	17.2%	13.7%	5.4%	10%
Male	9.7%	11.1%	6.1%	10.7%
25+				
Female	30.1%	27.6%	45.6%	32.6%
Male	5.4%	17%	9.5%	20.1%
Household size				
1–3 persons	31.2%	32.2%	51.7%	48%
4+ persons	68.8%	67.8%	48.3%	52%
No health insurance	34.6%		20.4%	
Medicaid/Childhealth Plus	42.3%		43.2%	
Person from household used home remedy in previous 12 months	56.1%		45.3%	

During meetings, residents identified more precisely some of the herbal mixtures and practices associated with home remedies than the survey data could provide. They also revealed that the folk medicinal practices were associated with spiritual beliefs such as *Santeria* and *Espiritismo* that are common among Caribbean Latinos from Puerto Rico, the Dominican Republic, and Cuba (Zayas and Ozuah 1996). According to community resident Neftali Rodriguez:

Look, everyone visits the *Botanica* for herbs and other remedies. I remember getting *empacho* as a kid [an illness of the gastrointestinal tract] and visiting a *santiguador* [herbal masseuse]. They [the *santiguadora*] would massage my stomach and put all these oils and spices and say all these prayers. It was all sort of weird as a kid, but we did it because that is what my *abuela* [grandmother] said would work!

One concern for the epidemiologists working with El Puente was that the home remedies might be toxic or exacerbating asthma attacks, and without more detailed information they could not make this determination (Ledogar 2000). While most herbal and home medicinal practices are not suspected of being harmful, at least one common practice, the use of metallic mercury, is suspected of causing serious health effects. Metallic mercury is sold in most *Botanicas* and is used for a number of religious healing practices. The mercury is sometimes worn around the neck, sprinkled in baby cribs, burned in candles, or ingested with wine to ward off evil spirits. Mercury is also ingested raw by some to relieve indigestion (Zayas and Ozuah 1996). El Puente was intent on engaging residents in discussions about home treatments to better understand what people were using for treatments and why they were so popular.

Practitioners of herbal treatments noted that the most common ingredients for treating asthma were lemon, aloe, anise, onion/shallot, and garlic, most of which were ingested with honey (Ledogar 2001b). These ingredients mostly were used as expectorants to rid someone of phlegm or to calm the airways (Iglesias-Garden 2001). Common mixtures used to prevent asthma attacks or treat someone experiencing an attack included oral doses of aloe, honey, and lemon; radish, onion, honey, and shark oil; and snake oil mixed with various herbs (Ledogar 2001b).

As the healers told their stories and explained what remedies they preferred for certain ailments, El Puente recorded these oral traditional practices. Since these recipes were being discussed and recorded in a public forum for the first time for many practitioners, the CHE workers were careful not to intervene too much when practitioners were telling their stories. According to Cecilia Iglesias-Garden:

For those of us in the Dominican community, it wasn't a surprise to hear about these home remedies. I think the use of snake oil, animal blood, boiled lizards, and owls meat, shocked the epidemiologists. But, we made sure not to allow the scientists to interrupt the women telling their stories. Even when the scientists wanted to butt-in or say that something might be harmful, or whatever, we didn't allow them to question the practices or methods, at first. Part of this was that we knew that these practices were not just about health, but also spiritual and religious. (Iglesias-Garden 2001)

According to Robert Ledogar of CIET, as the woman talked about their practices, it became obvious to the scientists that the use of home remedies could not be removed from their spiritual context. Ledogar noted that "this context often determined how and when the herbs were administered, how much was used, and the methods and frequency of ingestion. These were community traditions, not just health treatments" (Ledogar 2001).

Home Remedies and Pharmaceutical Medicine

The surveys also highlighted that residents not only relied on herbal and other culturally derived home remedies to treat asthma, but often used these in conjunction with and sometimes in place of physician-prescribed medication. However, specific questions were not asked about why residents were using home remedies to replace pharmaceutical medication. Thus, focus-group discussions were held to better understand this issue.

During CHE home visits with families and during community meetings, the outreach workers heard from many residents that they were regularly shunned and ridiculed by their health-care provider when they tried to explain their cultural or spiritual practices (Iglesias-Garden 2001). As a result, local people often did not trust physicians who made little or no effort to understand or appreciate their traditional and spiritual practices (Iglesias-Garden 2001). This sentiment was expressed to me by one resident:

Mira, I go to the doctor and he gives me two minutes of his time. He don't ask about whether I'm using some herbs. He don't really ask me nothin'. One time I say somethin' like, "Hey, I use this herb at home." He says, "Yeah, well do what you want, but that stuff don't work." I can't barely understand what he's sayin' most of the time anyways. Look, I just don't trust 'em 'cause they don't understand or even try to understand me.

El Puente learned that most residents using home remedies were not comfortable talking about their practices with their health-care provider and physicians were often insensitive to the role of cultural practices. According to Penchaszadeh of El Puente:

Because of trust, fear, and cultural issues, people were not telling their doctors about home remedies. The doctors were not asking them either. Since the doctors didn't relate to them, they wouldn't trust the medication they were giving them. Instead, they turned to what was comfortable—the home-remedies. (Penchaszadeh 2001)

This doctor-patient relationship and community resident's trust in prescribed medication also was reflected in the following story told to me by a high-school student at the El Puente Academy in Williamsburg:

Taking these [asthma] medications is a full time job. I got to do it three or more times a day, like taking a whole cocktail of stuff. It gets to be too much and sometimes I get lazy. I mean, like, I hate havin' to take 'em all the time, like a junky or sometin', right? Inhale this, pop this pill, where is my inhaler? It never fuckin' stops. The doctors tell me there are side effects. I feel 'em too, like I'm tired a lot, I be breakin' out, my face lookin' all busted. I even think they be makin' me gain weight, not sure 'dough. When I'm going out or somethin', you know on a date or to a party, shoot, I just say f—— it, no drugs for me. My doctor? He don't understand what its like taking all this shit. I mean it ain't all that bad, I mean, not bein' able to breathe is a lot worse, right? I mean, like, sometimes I just go to my *abuela* [grandmother] and have her give me some stuff. Her herbs, they be smelly and taste nasty, but its better than havin' to take all these drugs.

Accounts like these revealed that some residents not only did not trust their physicians and prefered traditional treatments, but that a physician-patient dialogue was crucial for effective asthma management. Without regular and candid discussion with a health-care provider, asthma sufferers were likely to avoid using medication and have trouble managing their condition. This finding helped El Puente plan interventions to improve this situation, including training physicians in cultural competency and having community members form teams of local people to collectively manage their asthma (Iglesias-Garden 2001).

Another survey finding about home remedies revealed that Dominicans were almost twice as likely to use home remedies as Puerto Ricans. During focus-group discussions Dominicans, who had more recently arrived in the neighborhood, spoke of being more disassociated from the health-care system than, for instance, their Puerto Rican neighbors. Dominican residents noted that home remedies were part and parcel of their familial and social networks, which often acted as their primary health-care system (Iglesias-Garden 2001). As one recent Dominican immigrant told me:

We came here from the DR [Dominican Republic] with nothing except friends and some family. These are the most important people who help you make it. I mean the government don't help and we didn't have any work. You do what you can and stay connected to your people—for jobs, food, a place to stay, and health care.

Thus, home remedies, especially for Dominicans, were more than just a source of health care; they were integral for staying connected to one's social network, which was crucial for daily survival and integration into American society. The importance of community networks for promoting health has been noted in Mexican American children who, despite having higher levels of poverty, lower levels of parental education, and more limited access to health care than non-Latino white children, have unexpectedly low rates of adverse perinatal outcomes and prevalence of chronic and disabling conditions (Mendoza and Fuentes-Afflick 1999).

The focus groups helped provide important contextual narratives to the quantitative survey data and revealed that for most Latinos, maintaining health was inseparable from the daily rhythms of everyday life. The community dialogues also instilled confidence in previously marginalized community members, particularly women, to speak about their expertise. Finally, listening to the explanations residents gave for some of the survey findings helped El Puente develop health-promoting interventions that resonated with local cultural practices.

Asthma Actions and Local Knowledge

The intention of El Puente's community-health project was not to gather local knowledge merely to challenge experts, but to improve the lives of neighborhood residents. Their approach was to organize residents for collective self-help. Self-help came in many forms. For example, after learning from the surveys that adults in the community also had severe asthma and that most adults did not know how to help children manage their asthma, the CHE developed a program called "asthma mastery in action" (Iglesias-Garden 2001).

The program developed individual asthma-management plans for adults, children, and families. The asthma-management program also enrolled residents without health insurance in a New York State free health-insurance program, ChildhealthPlus. The asthma-management plans are similar to daily diaries outlining where they travel and where they might encounter an asthma trigger in their daily activities. The management plans also asked questions about in-home triggers, such as housing condition, heating methods, smoking, pests/cockroaches, use of extermination chemicals, pets, typical humidity levels, and use of air filters, dehumidifiers, air conditioners, or other air regulators. The program was structured around a model for effective family- and individually focused asthma management, but also included collective disease management through the use of focus groups and programs to involve other community organizations and institutions in asthma awareness. The idea was to shift disease management from an often isolating and scary experience, especially when an asthma sufferer can not breathe, to a community-building experience.

The CHE team helped improve individual case management by doing such things as translating health documents, accompanying individuals to physicians' offices and helping patients understand their social service rights in legal hearings. The CHE team also facilitated the collective aspects of the asthma program by organizing group asthma-management sessions. Since many CHE workers were asthma sufferers or were taking care of family members with the disease, they were at once participants and facilitators of these community meetings (Iglesias-Garden 2001). El Puente's approach to asthma management involved learning, reflection, and actions in order to arrest the spread of the disease.[30]

Street Art and Asthma Awareness

Another action that grew out of some of the early community-survey work was a project by El Puente Academy students to raise community awareness about asthma. The students began a mural project depicting asthma's effects on individuals and the community, what might be causing and triggering the disease, and actions individuals and the community could take to address the disease. The mural covers the exposed wall of a three-story-high corner building in the heart of the community. It depicts some of the triggers of asthma (e.g., air pollution and cockroaches), what happens to the body during as asthma attack (e.g., red, inflamed lungs) and what sufferers can do for treatment (e.g., using inhalers, and women making herbal remedies) (figures 4.2 and 4.3).

Mural projects in urban neighborhoods have been called the "notebooks of the poor" (Barnett 1984). In many neighborhoods, walls are a place where the voiceless can tell their stories of anguish, injustice, and disease. But more than just recording their lives and struggles, murals are an effective way to communicate with the rest of the neighborhood, especially to youth. The neighborhood mural also has been used to alert local residents to the dangers of drugs, sexually transmitted diseases, and pollution. The student mural project translated the street science of local residents into street art and complemented the community surveys and dialogues.

Community Asthma Knowledge Influencing Professionals

While El Puente's focus has been to use local knowledge for collective self-help, community organizing, and capacity building within the neighborhood, their *street science* is also beginning to influence the practices of outsiders. After learning from residents that physicians often dismissed Latino folk medicinal practices in focus groups and that most residents avoided the local hospital, the CHE team developed a "cultural competency" training for local health-care providers. The training has CHE team members and other community residents educating health-care providers about Latino folk medicinal practices, including familial and spiritual aspects and the specific types of herbs and treatments residents commonly use (Iglesias-Garden 2001). The NYC DOH was considering using the El Puente trainings in other Latino neighborhoods around the city (Ledogar 2001).

The El Puente survey findings twice have been published in the *American Journal of Public Health*, suggesting that professional scien-

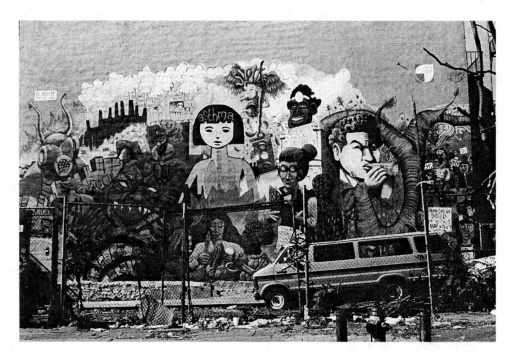

Figure 4.2.
El Puente asthma mural.

tists are taking note (Ledogar et al. 1999, 2000). One of the published findings from the El Puente work was that, to their surprise, the reported asthma period prevalence (e.g., persons reported as having been told by a doctor they have asthma and experience 1 or more asthma symptoms in the previous 12 months) was 5.3% among Dominicans and other Latinos and 13.2% among Puerto Ricans (Ledogar et al. 2000). This surprising finding could not be explained easily by residential location, household size, smoking, health insurance status, or educational attainment. This meant that Latinos living literally side-by-side were experiencing significantly different rates of asthma. This finding roused interest in El Puente's work by city agencies and academic researchers exploring explanations for differential disease rates among the diverse Latino population in the United States (Markides and Coreil 1986; Franzini, Ribble, and Keddie 2001).

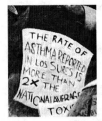
Epidemiology statistics

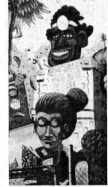
Medical care & education

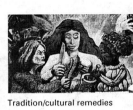
Tradition/cultural remedies

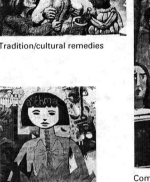
Community organizing

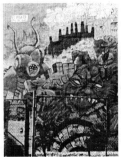
Air pollution exposures

Physiology

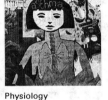

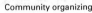

Figure 4.3.
Asthma mural: Some concepts.

El Puente's survey work also has been acknowledged by the National Institute of Environmental Health Sciences (NIEHS). The NIEHS has funded "The Williamsburg Brooklyn Asthma and Environment Consortium," which will establish El Puente as the principal investigator of a four-year community-based research partnership with Woodhull Medical and Mental Health Center and the New York University School of Medicine, Department of Environmental Medicine (NIEHS 2000). The NIEHS grant is aimed at addressing El Puente's original question that stimulated their first survey in 1995: What are the connections between asthma and environmental pollution? The grant will build on findings from some of El Puente's previous surveys, such as the importance of considering occupational health and workplace exposures, outdoor air-pollution monitoring, and indoor household-environmental assessments, to fully understand potential causes of local asthma (NIEHS 2000). According to the NIEHS, this project is unique because it will "document multiple exposures of residents in an industrial low-income community, use a community organizing model, focusing on capacity building of community residents through asthma self-help groups to conduct their own research, as well as design and implement interventions to improve environmental conditions" (NIEHS 2000).

While El Puente's *street science* was clearly influential in the neighborhood, it has had less impact on policy professionals. The strength of El Puente's *street science* was a direct result of the community organizing they did around asthma and community health generally. From the mobilization of students, to the hiring of community-health workers, to the focus-group meetings, the *street science* process for El Puente was as much about community organizing as data gathering. The group managed to gather persuasive narratives about the particular medicinal practices of residents, and they turned their findings into data publishable in one of the leading public-health journals in the country. However, this information did not lead to the passage of city-or statewide policy that might have targeted resources toward fighting the inner-city asthma epidemic.

El Puente's *street science* clearly aimed to extend, but not replace, conventional science. Augmenting traditional epidemiological survey methods and analysis tools with local insights and community participation, the group managed to alter a professional practice to better align with community priorities, knowledge, and ideology. The work improved on the science that outsiders could have directed. For instance, the group did not just document new and unexpected findings, such as the elevated asthma rates for older women and the different disease rates among Dominicans and Puerto Ricans, but they highlighted the meanings and potential causes associated with these findings. Professional epidemiologists rarely are concerned with this aspect of surveys, largely because they are rewarded for interesting quantitative findings, not the subjective understandings that give life to the numbers.

An important factor that may have limited the influence of El Puente's street science on professional decision making was that El Puente's efforts were not linked to a larger social movement. While the group initially tried to build a community-wide coalition to perform an asthma survey, that effort failed. The group also chose not to align itself with other groups in NYC that were conducting asthma research, such as The Point Community Development Corporation in the Bronx or West Harlem Environmental Action (Claudio 1996; Corbin-Mark 2001). One reason these community-based organizations did not partner was that they were all competing for the same private-foundation and government-sponsored grants. While El Puente eventually received the NIEHS grant to continue its asthma work, other community groups, particularly those in G/W, did not. Funding competition led to isolation and the failure to mobilize a city-wide asthma coalition.

A second reason El Puente may not have linked its *street science* to the national movement for childhood asthma prevention is that no such organized movement exists. The lack of a federally directed effort to monitor and address asthma was raised by the Pew Environmental Health Coalition in a recent study of the nationwide asthma epidemic (Pew 2000). The environmental-justice movement only recently has made asthma the focus of its organizing efforts. At a 2000 National Environmental Justice Advisory Committee meeting held to discuss environmental health, no sessions were dedicated solely to discussing the asthma epidemic in communities of color (NEJAC 2001). The attention given to asthma differs markedly from that given to other epidemic diseases, such as HIV/AIDS. In the case of AIDS research discussed in chapter 2, activists mobilized to challenge government research protocols and began performing their own biomedical research. Clearly, the "constituency" for asthma is mostly children of the urban poor and people of color, not the largely white, well-off organizers of the AIDS movement (Epstein 1996). In the absence of a national "asthma movement," the influence of El Puente's work remained largely neighborhood-focused.

Content with using its research for "community self-help," El Puente partnered with intermediaries to perform its street science but not to promote its findings in the larger policymaking community. Robert Ledogar, the epidemiologist from CIET, helped the group engage with professional research methods. While Ledogar acted as the lead author on the *AJPH* publications, the CHE team collected the survey data, and some assisted with the surveys' statistical analyses. When El Puente presented its work outside the neighborhood, Ledogar was always joined by Analia Penchaszadeh, the director of El Puente's Environmental Health and Justice Programs, Cecilia Iglesias-Garden, the coordinator of the CHE, and Luis Garden-Acosta, executive director of El Puente (Ledogar 2001).

Finally, El Puente's *street science* was successful because the group was able to identify and implement acute disease-management interventions without losing their interest in exploring the structural forces that might be causing the disease. The group's asthma-management program capitalized on funding from the City to improve asthma treatment for disease sufferers and their families, while El Puente's focus-group discussions explored potential economic and social determinants of the disease, such as access to quality health care, immigration policies, occupational flexibility, and environmental exposures. In addition, evaluations of the home environment performed as part of the CHE asthma-management plan, helped highlight the role of housing quality and affordability for understanding the asthma puzzle in urban neighborhoods. Finally, the community health workers' door-to-door outreach work revealed that for families in the neighborhood, like those in other impoverished urban communities, asthma is just one of a panoply of overlapping health and well-being issues that they struggle with on a daily basis, but a disease that causes significant disruption to regular family, school, and workplace participation.

While El Puente's *street science* may not have had a direct influence on professional actions outside the neighborhood, community knowledge played an integral role in highlighting and implementing strategies to address asthma in the Latino community. The *street science* process also acted to organize community members—a success that professionals should not overlook. If professionals are to work well with residents, they must understand what residents claim to know and how working together can improve the health of disadvantaged groups. This case highlighted that *street science* helps community organizations learn and build trust and credibility with both local residents and outside professionals, and that that these qualities are crucial for effective partnerships aimed at eliminating persistent chronic diseases such as asthma.

5

Lead Poisoning and the Discourse of Local Knowledge

Finally, we have arrived at the age of extreme specialization, the present age, when the amount of specialized knowledge, often accurate, often extremely refined, has far outstripped our capacity to make use of it as part of a consistent whole. The remedy for this is not to be found in any mechanical combination of specialisms. . . . The cure lies rather in starting from the common whole—a region, its activities, its people, its configuration, its total life—and relating each further achievement in specialized knowledge to this cluster of images and experiences.

—Lewis Mumford, *Culture of Cities*

Cari Comart watched as flakes fell into her yard and windows. The flakes weren't snow; it was June after all. The flakes were paint chips from sandblasting work on the Williamsburg Bridge 200 feet away from her home. She shut her windows and called her neighbors. After learning that that the paint was lead-based, she brought her 18-month-old daughter Bettina to a physician. Bettina's blood-lead levels were 4 times the levels deemed safe by the health department. Comart then had the soil in her yard tested, and the samples came back with readings 4,000 times above acceptable limits.

Comart heard similar stories of lead poisoning coming from her neighbors. She helped organize residents and they filed a lawsuit against the Department of Transportation (DOT), to stop the sandblasting being performed in preparation for bridge repainting. The lawsuit, however, would not be heard quickly enough for some parents, so they filed for a court-ordered injunction to stop the bridge work immediately. They also demanded that the City begin testing neighborhood children and soil. Within weeks, construction was stopped and New York City officials confirmed that nearly 100 soil samples around the bridge had indeed exceeded 1,000 parts per million (ppm). At one spot in Williamsburg, the City found a reading of 42,096 ppm.

Responding to pressure from residents, who had gained the support of the media and politicians, the city agreed to test and remediate soil around the bridge. While the City agreed to the actions, they insisted that the elevated lead levels in soils were not a result of the bridge sandblasting, but rather from historic lead deposits from leaded gasoline and the widespread use of lead paint on and inside of older homes. Weeks passed and the City's promises went unfulfilled. Sandblasting restarted before soil and blood tests were performed.

The community returned to the judge and asked for a court order to stop the work again. Before the court ruled, the City agreed to form a mayoral task force to devise new procedures for sandblasting on city bridges, including the Williamsburg Bridge. The task force met for over a year, and in 1994, two years after the first paint chips fell into Comart's yard, the task force issued new guidelines for bridge paint removal that they claimed would be protective of human health and the environment. The community, however, did not trust the guidelines, even though some community members had been members of the task force. The community sued the City again, claiming this time that the recommendations should be required to undergo a full environmental review and be subject to public hearings and comment. The City disagreed. Sandblasting restarted on the Williamsburg Bridge, this time with the City following the guidelines recommended by the task force. The community pursued its case to the New York State Supreme Court, and in November 1996, the court ruled that the City must cease all sandblasting and perform an environmental and public-health review of the work.

This chapter discusses how the community organized its street science to support its legal claims and convinced the city to prepare an environmental impact statement (EIS). Part of the final settlement between the community and the City was that the EIS would include a public-health assessment, and the City agreed to provide financial assistance to the community to hire its own professionals to assist them in reviewing the risk assessment. This chapter highlights the challenges the community coalition faced during interactions with its own professional consultants, particularly as residents and experts clashed over the most effective methods for community input into the EIS and health assessment. In particular, it highlights the face-to-face interactions during these meetings between professional outsiders hired by locals and the locals themselves. Through an account of the communication challenges community residents often face when talking with professionals, the chapter highlights some typical challenges facing *street science* when discourse forums are limited to those defined by professionals.

Analyzing Community Discourse

The discourse between professionals and community members raises many challenges when local people are forced to frame street science in the language of professional science. Even when we all speak the same language, interaction is not an unproblematic simple exchange of fact and opinion, and obtaining and relaying information is thus a social, not a technical, problem (Habermas 1990). Important aspects of community power relations are masked in public communicative encounters. Urban planners are the professionals often thrust into contentious community dialogues, and the field has struggled with how to manage issues of culture, power, conflict, and the legitimacy of the planner's role in these situations for much of the past four decades (Peattie 1968; Arnstein 1969; Benveniste 1972; Kemp 1985; Forester 1989; Amy 1987; Healey 1997; Susskind et al. 1999). While recent work in planning tends to celebrate community victories over indifferent developers and local governments and highlights the strategies that shaped those victories (e.g., Medoff and Sklar 1994), less attention is being paid to how planners ought to reconceptualize their practice to effectively manage the economic, political, and cultural dimensions of science-intensive disputes.[31] Some analyses have helped professionals understand why certain public processes fail and others succeed. For example, Tauxe (1995), in a study of a development process in western North Dakota, shows how community voices were marginalized by planners who attended more closely to technical styles of discourse. Community voices were marginalized despite public efforts to involve residents. Even when local residents managed to gain an audience, they had little impact on development decisions in part because planners and residents did not speak the same language and understand each other's politics (Tauxe 1995). Planners failed to see their role as mediators and bridge-builders (Susskind and Cruikshank 1987).

These findings are common in the planning literature, particularly in analyses of environmental-health disputes. For example, in a study of public meetings around one of the nation's largest toxic-waste disposal sites, Kaminstein found that public officials overwhelmed local residents with technical data, responded to anxious inquiries with confusing scientific explanations, and in trying to validate residents' concerns as important and understandable, often came across to the audience as arrogant, aloof, and patronizing (1996, 461). Lowry, Adler, and Milner, in a study of citizen involvement in planning in Hawaii, found that public deliberations often fail when planners "regard meeting facilitation as merely a set of techniques to be acquired, mastered, and applied as part of the planner's skill kit" (1997, 186). They argue that successful meeting facilitation requires planners to understand the political power dynamics inherent in group processes, such as who facilitates meetings, who sponsors the facilitators, who is invited, how decisions will be made, and how generated information will be used.

The conflict between the City and the residents of G/W over the sandblasting of leaded paint from the Williamsburg Bridge highlights the "micro-deliberative politics" of street science. The account reveals the historical context within which community residents enter into discourse with professionals. The historical review is also crucial for understanding the experiential knowledge and street science that locals bring into the health-impact-analysis process. Then the chapter zooms in on the face-to-face discourse between a community coalition and the professionals the coalition hired to help them navigate through the environmental-impact statement and accompanying public-health assessment of the bridge work. A retelling of community meetings, coupled with interviews of the participants reflecting on the encounters, shows some of the challenges professionals and community members face during face-to-face dialogues that seek to include *street science* in decision making.

Community Discovery and Coalition Building

In June of 1992, the DOT sandblasting work on the Williamsburg Bridge began, with no prior environmental review. According to Joe Ketas, NYC DEP assistant commissioner, the work was considered routine maintenance and improvements, which by law do not require a full environmental review. The blasting caused dust clouds that showered an area around the bridge of at least 10 square blocks. According to Inez Pasher, who lived one block from where the blasting took place:

It was like pin pricks when you got hit by the dust. It should have been captured by tarps, but it wasn't. That dust was constantly moving around. It was horrible. It moved inside on your clothes and through windows. (Pasher 2001)

Pasher, a Latina who describes herself as a "self-taught environmentalist," collected dust samples in her home. She went to her neighbors' doors and asked them to do the same. She described her actions that day:

I went around, door-to-door, and asked who noticed the dust and whether it was giving them a problem. We collected dust samples from inside and outside homes. We also took some soil samples in yards and playgrounds right around the bridge. We called the City DOT and State DEC to complain. (Pasher 2001)

Inez and her neighbors collected approximately 15 grams of debris from their windowsills and from the top of a table in a backyard garden (Mitchell 1992a). They also videotaped the dust clouds from the bridge blasting as they settled on the neighborhood, playgrounds, and their own yards. On June 15, 1992, they sent the samples to a lab in New Jersey.[32] According to Cari Comart, Pasher's neighbor:

When I called the lab later that week, I was told that the samples contained 4.57% per weight lead, or 45,700 parts per million. I was advised by the lab, in no uncertain terms, that the lead levels were extremely dangerous and should be corrected as soon as possible. (Mitchell 1992b)

The work of these residents was inquiry, knowledge production, and organizing all at once. It also suggests a rational order to community mobilization of local health knowledge when something new and suspicious is discovered. Brown and Mikkelsen (1990) note that community residents often begin with observations, hypothesize connections between what they observe and adverse health, contact professionals for answers, and then organize others into a coalition.[33] This early work by Pasher galvanized both community and professional attention to lead poisoning in the community.

On June 17, 1992, inspectors from numerous City and State agencies visited Pasher and witnessed for themselves the clouds of lead-based paint from the sandblasting operation. By 3 p.m. that day, the NYS DEC shut down the sandblasting operation due to the contractor's inability to contain emissions of blasted paint. However, operations continued sporadically until July 8, when the State issued a court order ceasing the operations (NYC DOT 1998).

Test results taken from soil around the bridge by the NYC DOH when inspectors visited in June revealed elevated levels of lead, with all readings exceeding 1,000 ppm and one sample over 42,000 ppm. Children whose blood was tested weeks after the incident were found to have blood-lead levels exceeding city- and federal-action levels. Many readings were between 15 and 20 µg/dl of lead in the blood, while the actionable levels are 10 µg/dl (NYC DOT 1998).[34]

The City reacted to the sampling and blood-lead tests by vacuum cleaning the surrounding streets. Rooftops, sidewalks, streets, and playgrounds also were scheduled to be swept. During this period, the NYC DEP ruled that readings equal to or less than 1,000 ppm were normal urban background conditions.[35] Dr. Andrew Goodman, the assistant commissioner for the NYC DOH, said at the time that the department was concerned about the "very high levels of lead," but that such levels were not unexpected in New York, as in most urban centers, where decades of automobile exhaust and paint flaking from buildings and bridges had tainted soil. "Our assessment is that these are levels that most likely have been around for a long period of time," Goodman said. "These are levels of great concern, but in fact the threat is not that significant because there are very few children playing in the streets directly beneath the bridges" (quoted in Myers 1992c). But community leaders did not see it the same way, according to Luis Garden-Acosta, executive director of El Puente: "We're in the middle of a modern-day Love Canal, and we can't act as business as usual. We're dealing with a lead emergency and our community is being held hostage" (quoted in Holloway 1994).

Pasher organized residents and local groups into a coalition to sue the City so that the bridge work would be halted immediately and soil remediation and blood screening would take place to determine the impact of the sandblasting on local residents' health. A group called the Williamsburg Around the Bridge Block Association (WABBA) formed and included representatives from local organizations such as Community Board 1, El Puente, UJO, and the Watchperson Project. The group also included organizations from outside the community, such as the South Bronx Clean Air Coalition and the New York City Coalition to End Lead Poisoning, that were concerned about the impacts of lead paint in other neighborhoods. Pasher was able to organize WABBA by sharing her experience of the lead flakes falling from the bridge sandblasting into her home and the resulting tests that showed extremely elevated concentrations of lead with other organizations. She capitalized on media attention to the issue and used her position as a member of the environmental committee of the local community board (a neighborhood planning council) to mobilize activists to form WABBA (Myers 1992a).

WABBA demanded that the City halt the bridge work and assess the health and environmental impacts of the work. As the pressure mounted, NYC Mayor Dinkins decided to convene a mayoral-level task force to review bridge-painting procedures city wide. The task force, charged with developing new protocols for bridge work and addressing the lead-paint exposures and health concerns in the Williamsburg community, consisted of city- and state-level agencies, the U.S. EPA, elected officials, technical and medical professionals, and community representatives (Myers 1992a). The bridge repainting task force also was charged with drafting procedures to respond to WABBA's environmental and health concerns, as well as recommendations for how the City could proceed effectively and safely with the bridge work.

A year and a half later, the Task Force had devised new protocols. The City adopted these new guidelines for repainting work on all 838 city bridges. The Task Force worked quickly because the bridge work was $30 million over budget after the almost-two-year delay (Dube 1994). The Task Force guidelines were reviewed and approved by the U.S. EPA, and the state DEC and DOH (Ketas 1999). The procedures included protocols for containment of sandblasted paint, continuous soil and air monitoring during bridge work, cleanup protocols for existing contaminated soil and community-notification procedures for lead-paint-removal operations. The Task Force recommended that all sandblasting be fully contained in negative-air-pressure tents, that real-time air monitoring occur and ambient-air and soil monitoring be performed periodically. The protocol also required that work be halted when a number of thresholds were violated (NYC DOT 1998).

WABBA rejected the Task Force's findings. Comart, one of the community representatives on the task force, noted that "the protocols were not protective of human health and virtually gave the city a green-light to poison more people with lead paint" (quoted in Dube 1994). She also stated that the task force ran roughshod over citizen concerns and adopted guidelines to suit the City's concerns, not WABBA. While the community agreed that the protocols were an improvement on the procedures the City had started with, WABBA chose to sue the City anyway because they feared the protocols would not be strictly enforced. According to Manfred Hecht, a community resident and member of both the task force and WABBA:

The monitoring of these procedures is being thrown completely into the contractors' hands, which is suicide. We want to make sure there are effective checks and balances in place. We don't know if what we came up with at the table is safe. We [the community members] didn't have the expertise. (quoted in Dube 1994)

Within weeks of the City's announcement that they had formed a city-wide consensus for new, protective protocols for bridge-repainting work, WABBA filed suit. The community suit claimed that since the task force had devised new rules that were in effect new regulations, the protocols must be subject to city and state environmental and public-review requirements. The City denied this and restarted the sandblasting work on the bridge before the lawsuit could be heard in court. WABBA went immediately to the judge, demanding a stay on all work until the City could show that lead paint from the sandblasting did not pose a threat to human health (Van Natta 1995).

Community knowledge was instrumental in creating WABBA and the lawsuit. The coalition gathered the stories of numerous residents in order to tell a passionate narrative about a dangerous and involuntary exposure. These stories helped mobilize and broaden WABBA's support. Community narratives of the paint flakes falling in the streets, the results of some blood-lead tests from children living near the bridge, and local accounts of delay or inaction by the City in response to local concerns formed the basis of the legal claim, which also built on the city's history of lead-poisoning politics (Van Natta 1995).

Lead Poisoning in New York City

Lead is a poisonous heavy metal that often is found in old paint, old pipes, and other industrial materials. Lead particles that enter the human body cause severe damage to the brain and central nervous system. Children who have absorbed lead can suffer impaired intellectual development, shortened attention spans, and behavioral disorders, and/or anemia and impaired metabolism of vitamin D (Schwartz 1994). Much of this damage is permanent and irreversible. Children from birth through 6 years old have the highest risk of lead poisoning. Their normal hand-to-mouth activity causes more frequent ingestion of contaminated particles. More significantly, children's brains and nervous systems are particularly vulnerable in their early developmental stages. Children also are more vulnerable to lead poisoning because they retain two times more of the lead that they ingest than adults. During the period of greatest risk for lead poisoning, when children are 9–18 months old, they absorb lead at a rate that is 5 to 10 times higher than adults (Ruff et al. 1996). In addition, because their bodies are smaller, a smaller amount of ingested or inhaled lead can result in a higher concentration in a child than in an adult (ATSDR 1988; Silbergeld 1997).

Over the past 20 years, childhood lead poisoning has declined dramatically in the United States due to limits on lead in gasoline, paint, food cans, and other consumer products. While lead poisoning crosses all socioeconomic, geographic, and racial boundaries, the burden of this disease falls disproportionately on low-income families and families of color. In the United States, children from poor families are 8 times more likely to be poisoned than those from higher-income families (CDC 1991). African-American children are 5 times more likely to be poisoned than white children. Nationwide, about 22% of African-American children living in older housing are lead poisoned (ATSDR 1988). According to the Agency for Toxic Substances Disease Registry (ATSDR), 88% of all children with family incomes below $6,000—80.4% of whites and

96.5% of African-Americans—are estimated to be affected by lead poisoning. While the total number of NYC children documented with blood-lead levels at or above 20 µg/dl in 1995 was 2,727, the number of children in the city under age 6 with blood-lead levels documented at or above 10 µg/dl during this same year was 18,728—nearly 7 times higher. (For all children below 18 years old, the total is 21,158) (Green 1998, 17). The NYC DOH estimates that in 1995, approximately 35,000 children under 6 years old in the city had blood lead levels of 10 µg/dl or higher.

Under normal conditions, or what might be considered the background conditions in New York City, children are expected to have no more than 2.7 µg/dl of lead in their blood. In the city, the DOH commonly uses the term "lead poisoning case" to refer to those instances in which it must inspect a child's dwelling and order abatement of lead-based paint hazards—which is required when a child has a blood lead level of 10 µg/dl or more. The city's health code defines the condition of "lead poisoning" as occurring at a blood-lead level of 10 µg/dl or higher.[36] This level is consistent with the guidelines of the federal Centers for Disease Control, which made the "action level" for lead in children's blood more stringent in 1991 by reducing the level from 25 to 10 µg/dl, urging close monitoring of any child whose blood-lead level is within the range of 10–14 µg/dl, and requiring further action if it rises above that level (Landrigan 2000).

Although New York City was one of the first jurisdictions to ban the sale of lead paint (in 1960; most of the rest of the country didn't ban lead paint until 1978), lead paint remains pervasive; the vast majority of painted structures constructed before 1960 contain some lead paint. The 1990 Census indicated that New York City has the nation's highest percentage of pre-1960 residential housing (63.5%). The City estimates that almost 2 million units of housing have lead-based paint, approximately half of which are occupied by persons of low or moderate income; an estimated 323,000 apartments with lead paint have young children residing there, and of these, some 174,000 are occupied by low-income families (Green 1998).

Until 1982, the City could demand the removal of lead paint only after a child was already poisoned. However, lead poisoning is a permanent injury, so waiting until a child is poisoned is too late. In 1982, the City enacted Local Law 1, which required landlords to remove lead paint immediately in any multiple dwelling where there were young children. The law was one of the strongest lead poisoning prevention laws in the country but the City never enforced it fully (Green 1998).

In 1985, the New York City Coalition to End Lead Poisoning (NYC-CELP) brought a class-action suit against the City that resulted in several court orders directing the City to fully enforce Local Law 1. In 1996, the state Court of Appeals declared that under Local Law 1 landlords had a continuing obligation to ensure that dwellings with young children were free of lead hazards. However, in 1999 the City Council rolled back the lead-poisoning laws by enacting Local Law 38, despite the virtually universal objections of public-health professionals; physicians; tenant organizations; disability, education, and environmental groups; racial-justice organizations; and labor unions (Green 1998).

Local Law 38 shifted much of the burden of detecting and responding to lead hazards from landlords to tenants, eliminated from regulatory control lead dust (generally considered the prime cause of lead poisoning), and scaled back the safety measures and training required during lead-removal work (Green 1998). Subsequently, NYCCELP and other organizations sued the City again, this time asserting that the City Council violated state law by enacting Local Law 38 without a proper environmental review. The state Supreme Court agreed, in October 2000 declaring Local Law 38 null and void and reinstating Local Law 1 (Lambert 2000).

The Community's Case against the Bridge Sandblasting

In building its case against the bridge sandblasting, WABBA used many of the same arguments that were successful in overturning Local Law 38. In fact, the NYCCELP was a party to both cases and helped argue that any new rules should undergo a comprehensive environmental review (DOT 1998). In WABBA's case, the community coalition rejected the task force's guidelines, insisting that in addition to failing to perform adequate environmental and public-notification reviews, the task force failed to address existing lead poisoning in the Williamsburg neighborhood. Citing the NYC DOH blood screening in which 712 children between 1 and 6 years old were tested and 95 had blood-lead levels above 10 µg/dl and 7 above 20 µg/dl, WABBA demanded that the City address existing health hazards. According to Annemarie Crocetti, an epidemiologist who attended the task force meetings and assisted the community in its lawsuit, the task force was designed from the outset to support what the City wanted. She noted in an affidavit:

As far as I know, and I attended almost every Task Force meeting, there were no motions proposed, seconded, amended or voted on. The minutes do not necessarily represent the Task Force consensus of what took place at the meetings. The Task Force Chair and other city officials failed to pay serious and meaningful attention to the comments, objections, criticisms expressed by community members of the Task Force. (Crocetti 1994, 3)

In building its case against the City, WABBA relied heavily on John Rosen, a professor of pediatrics, head of the Division of Environmental Sciences at Albert Einstein College of Medicine, and an attending physician at Montefiore Medical Center in the Bronx. In his affidavit submitted with the community's lawsuit, Rosen noted that "compared to lead from peeling paint in residential housing, the concentration of lead from lead painted bridges is many orders of magnitude higher in lead content" (Rosen 1994, 8). The WABBA case claimed the work of the task force was inadequate, not entirely due to the new guidelines, but because the group failed to address remediation, monitoring and health-screening concerns of the community, including:[37]

1) Remediation

a) Failure to conduct a systematic survey of the extent of lead contamination in the neighborhood.

b) Failure to obtain soil samples from residential areas, including yards and gardens.

c) Failure to take interior household dust samples and measure them for lead.

d) Remediation efforts have been ad hoc and, without the aforementioned sampling data, misguided. For example, the city tested in concentric zones around the bridge in 1/10th of a mile increments (500 feet). The percentage of samples found to have lead contamination in excess of 1,000 ppm in zones 1–5 were 84.6%, 42.1%, 16.2%, 33.3%, and 34.8%, respectively. Yet, the city only performed remediation in zone 1.

2) Public Health Screening

e) Determination that neighborhood children were "safe" was based on blood samples taken 3 months after the sandblasting event, and no follow-up sampling has occurred to confirm that lead levels have decreased.

f) The NYC DOH failed to institute an "intensive blood-lead monitoring program," relying instead on testing of only children of residents who "complained."

3) Monitoring

g) The task force protocols give no detail about how and how often the paint removal procedures will be "continuously analyzed to ensure their safety and efficiency" nor do they specify which agency will be responsible for these analyses. Additionally, the task force protocols do not define what standards, health or environmental, will be used "to determine the effectiveness of these operations."

h) The protocols do not specify what standard will be used for the continuous air monitoring and "visible inspections." The protocols fail to specify how and by whom waste paint will be disposed. The protocols rely on city agencies and community organizations to notify residents of a violation, but there is no requirement for the city to notify residents directly or through local physicians, hospitals, clinics, or schools.

Based on these arguments, WABBA called for an immediate cessation of all bridge sandblasting and for an environmental impact assessment to be performed by the City. In addition, they recommended that an independent body of multidisciplinary experts monitor the bridge-painting operations, to help ensure the safety and health of workers and the public. Using Pasher and Comart's videotape from the first few days of the sandblasting as part of their testimony, WABBA argued that the City was irresponsible and could not be trusted to oversee the work alone. The lawsuit claimed that "in light of the City's past record, the public should have little confidence that City officials will place health and safety over costs and efficiency." Finally, the group recommended that technological and engineering alternatives to sandblasting be explored and evaluated and, irregardless of the paint-removal technology chosen, "containment technology should be the most advanced and meet the highest engineering and safety standards" (Rosen 1994, 15).

Professional Response to Local Knowledge

Not surprisingly, the City rejected the claims made in the community's lawsuit and denied that the task force protocol would inadequately protect public health. According to Virginia Maher, an analyst with the mayor's Office of Operations and appointee to the task force, the community was correct in noting that the City "had no comprehensive set of procedures for lead paint removal prior to the development of the task force Protocol," but the task force "accomplished its goals by developing the bridge-work Protocol and a plan for blood lead screening of children living near the Williamsburg Bridge and for cleaning-up areas potentially affected by the release of lead dust from the abrasive blasting" (quoted in Stout 1996a).

Believing they had done enough with the task force protocols, the City resumed sandblasting on the bridge. However, State Supreme Court Justice Martin Schoenfeld ruled on October 6, 1995, that the City must halt operations on the bridge because the community's claims were valid. The judge ruled that the task force guidelines should have been subject to public hearings and an environmental review. In his decision, he wrote that the videotape shows "a dust cloud emanating from the work area on the bridge and what are arguably sloppy waste collection procedures."[38] The judge also stated that "there appears to have been a very good faith effort to draft a set of procedures that will minimize the escape of lead dust into the atmosphere, but I have neither the authority nor the expertise to judge the aforementioned procedures" (quoted in Stout 1996a).

Community knowledge played a role in WABBA's case convincing the Supreme Court that the City was negligent. The judge ruled for the community coalition largely based on numerous affidavits from residents describing the "careless sandblasting work" and the homemade video. The judge did not overturn the task force guidelines but merely agreed with the community that all of the City's work should be subject to a full environmental review.

The city appealed the ruling, and the appeals court refused an emergency motion from residents to stop the sandblasting work while the appeal was heard, so blasting started again (Van Natta 1995). Then, in June 1996, the Appellate Division of State Supreme Court ruled that the Supreme Court had ruled correctly in October 1995, halting the blasting and requiring an environmental impact statement and associated public hearings. "By all accounts," the appellate justices unanimously agreed, "the project was a public relations and public health fiasco" (quoted in Stout 1996a).

However, unclear wording of the appellate ruling left an opening for the City to continue work on the bridge. In its ruling, the appeals court had ordered the City either to conduct an environmental review or to issue a "negative declaration" ("NegDec"); that is, an assertion that the paint-removal work would have no significant environmental impacts and is exempt from an environmental review because, for example, the work is considered "normal maintenance." The community assumed that in order to issue a negative declaration, the City would have to perform some review to make the no-impact determination. However, the City interpreted the ruling as *either* an environmental review *or* a negative declaration. Since the City had already issued a "NegDec" when it approved the bridge work in 1992, they interpreted the Court's ruling as a green light for them to resume sandblasting, which they did in the summer of 1996 (Stout 1996b).

The community, thinking they had won the case, was shocked to see sandblasting operations resuming on the bridge (George 1996). WABBA returned to the appeals court in July, as the work on the bridge continued, to ask that the language of the June ruling be clarified. The justices agreed to review the language but did not halt the sandblasting. Finally, in October the Appellate Division issued a revised decree clarifying the June ruling. The decree halted sandblasting on the Williamsburg Bridge only and required the City to comply with state environmental review requirements. The City contemplated an appeal for a month and then, on November 7, entered into a Stipulation of Settlement ending the lawsuit and ending the City's right to appeal. The community continued to argue that the bridge work presented a health risk to local children, while the City stated that they agreed to the EIS because, according to Jane Earle, assistant corporation council for the city, "it looked like that would be the fastest way for us to get back to work" (quoted in Stout 1996b). In the settlement, the City agreed to perform an environmental impact assessment that included a public-health analysis (they refused to call it a risk assessment) and hold all required public hearings. A key piece of the settlement was that the City must finance WABBA to hire experts of its own choosing to help them comment on and participate in the EIS and public-health analyses.

Community Discourse about the Environmental Impact Statement

In the EIS, the City tried to be clear that the public-health assessment should not be considered a typical risk assessment.

A public health assessment done as part of an EIS differs from the more common use of risk assessment to evaluate sites requiring remediation. As described in the Introduction to this EIS, the purpose of an EIS is to evaluate a set of future actions, including the "no action" alternative, in terms of a defined goal or objective. While it is necessary to understand existing conditions, a complete analysis of conditions or quantification of environmental conditions that produced the existing public health conditions is not necessary to an EIS. This differs from a risk assessment conducted, for example, at a Superfund site, where the goal of the risk assessment is to identify present conditions that cause current or future public health threats, and recommend remediation goals. An EIS does not assess current conditions or develop remediation goals. (DOT 1998, 10-1)

The community, however, was under a different impression. The group called a series of meetings both to understand the different aspects of the EIS and to formulate a coalition position. The group enlisted the support of two lead-poisoning experts from Mt. Sinai School of Medicine, Nancy Clark and Steven Levin, to assist them with the technical review of the public-health assessment. From the outset WABBA seemed fractured over the selection and use of the outside experts. Some members were grateful for the help while a vocal minority expressed distrust of the Mt. Sinai experts. The internal group tension eventually led to the dismissal of the Mt. Sinai experts and the hiring of new consultants. The group would hire Berger, Lehman Associates, P.C. (BLA) who later subcontracted with the Hunter College Center for Occupational and Environmental Health. The key contact person at Hunter was Daniel Kass, director of the COEH and someone with a history of working with community organizations in G/W. Kass had helped the community convince the DEP in 1991 to fund the first health study of the neighborhood through the Environmental Benefits Program. Under Kass's direction, the center also helped the

Watchperson Project participate in the BAEL project and worked with the Watchperson Project to develop their own geographic information system (GIS) (Kass 2001). Kass also had volunteered to conduct trainings in epidemiology for El Puente's community-health workers. In short, Kass was a knowledgeable, recognized, and respected public-health professional in the eyes of most community members working on environmental health issues, and unlike the Mt. Sinai experts, he was trusted by all WABBA members (Swanston 1999).

The draft EIS concluded that since the DOT would institute new containment procedures for the abrasive sandblasting work on the bridge, the work would create no significant additional health risk of lead poisoning. Since the proposed paint-removal procedures would not result in the release of significant amounts of fugitive materials (lead paint dust particles) into the surrounding environment, increases to blood-lead levels also would be not significant. Even under the worst-case scenario, which the City determined to be the "no action alternative" because lead paint would "flake-off in an uncontrolled manner due to weathering and deterioration," no significant blood-lead increases would occur (DOT 1998, S-15).[39] Some of the key public health assessment conclusions included:

1. Blood-lead levels studied on both sides of the Williamsburg Bridge were not related to proximity to the bridge.[40]

2. Maximum worst-case scenario releases without mitigation were projected to result in a long-term increase in child blood-lead levels of 1.14 μg/dl for 0–1 year olds, 1.6 μg/dl for 1–3 year olds, 0.98 μg/dl for 2–3 year olds, 0.85 μg/dl for 3–4 year olds, 0.53 μg/dl for 4–5 year olds, and 0.43 μg/dl for 5–6 year olds.

3. Maximum worst case scenario releases without mitigation would result, among children most exposed, in a long-term increase in the percent of children considered "lead poisoned" (>20 μg/dl) by a maximum of 1.3%, but generally by about 0.1%.

4. Short-term increases in child blood-lead levels resulting from unmitigated maximum worst-case release scenarios are far greater than projected long-term changes, as is the percent of children whose blood-lead levels would be elevated to the point requiring immediate medical attention (45 μg/dl).

The City's Lead-Exposure Models

The City arrived at their conclusions after modeling potential lead exposure and uptake. They used three EPA models to estimate the probability
of community lead exposures and human uptake of lead. One model,
called the Integrated Exposure Uptake Biokinetic (IEUBK) model, normally was used for estimating blood-lead uptake from lead-paint exposure in the home and for designing remedial action in a home, a building,
or an area as large as a city block. The second model, called Bower et al.,
was used for estimating lead releases and dispersion rates from bridge
work (DOT 1998, 10-2). The IEUBK model estimates steady-state blood-
lead levels reflecting exposure to lead in multiple media (diet, drinking
water, air, soil, and dust) over an extended period of time, and the City
chose a 25-year period to model exposures. A third model, called the
O'Flaherty Model, was used to estimate short-term acute exposures and
their impact on blood lead levels in both children and adults.

The IEUBK model used data inputs from the NYC DOH, which
recorded blood-lead measurements from children around the city aged
0–6 years old. The model used over 56,000 individual blood-lead measurements for model inputs representing, according to the City, a spa-
tially and demographically representative sample of city children (DOT
1998, S-12). These data acted as the blood-level baselines for children,
and the model estimated the likely uptake of lead for all children around
bridges, including those in Williamsburg. For adults, the Bowers et al.
model used blood-lead data from the National Health and Nutrition
Examination Survey (DOT 1998, 10-2).

Both models generate probabilities of lead uptake based on a known
exposure. However, the City claimed that they did not have accurate
lead-emissions information from sandblasting, so the EIS ran the risk
models "backward." In other words, the EIS started the models by
inputting estimated blood-lead levels in children (based on the data
described above), modeled an increase in blood lead to "safe levels" (10
µg/dl was chosen as the default value), and then, based on these two estimates, the model generated the concentrations of lead in different media
(air, soil, water, etc.) that would be admissible for blood-lead to remain
under the "safe levels." The City claimed that using the models this way,

while unconventional, would generate overly conservative lead-emissions requirements (DOT 1998, 10-2, 4).

In addition, the EIS stipulated that the bridge sandblasting would be contained in a sheath and the "stringency of containment" would be based on the proximity of bridge work to residences. In industrial areas the containment would be less strict than in residential areas. Finally, an environmental consultant would be hired to monitor all lead-paint-removal activities, would be under the direction of the NYC DOT, and would be instructed to inform the City of any violation of containment procedures.

Debating Whose Evidence Should Count

The community reacted to the EIS by holding a meeting with WABBA and its new consultant. The consultant, Kass from Hunter College, joined a community group already fractured over the dismissal of the first experts from Mt. Sinai and because of other political battles operating in parallel to the review of the EIS.[41] WABBA met a number of times with Kass, who helped walk the community members through the EIS, the health assessment, and the implications of the findings.[42] During one WABBA meeting in July 1998, Kass led the discussion, beginning by reviewing a memo that he had written to the group summarizing key findings of the draft EIS. From the outset, Kass noted that the findings were "not good" and that the risk assessment had revealed little new information about potential risks. Kass suggested that the group might not want to get "bogged down" in the messy science of the health assessment and instead might concentrate on the monitoring and public-notification aspects of the EIS. He reminded the group that the monitoring and procedural issues were most convincing for the judge and led to the order for the city to perform the EIS in the first place (Kass 1999).

There was an awkward silence before some residents began leaning over and whispering to one another. "We came here to find out if our kids are at risk. Do you know what it is like to have a lead poisoned child?" shouted someone in the group. Kass acknowledged the concern and affirmed their worries: "I have the same concerns as you do." And, he added, the best way to ensure that local kids are safe is to press the

City to do the work properly and get them to allow residents to monitor and stop the work if any apparent violations occur. Again, he did not suggest that the group should challenge the lead-exposure findings.

According to Samara Swanston, "The process was designed up front to ensure their [the City's] scenario was the only viable alternative." A Latina from the Caribbean asked why the group wasn't "focusing on the real issue; lead poisoning and whether the work should go ahead at all."[43] Her comment immediately shifted the focus of the meeting. Heads in the group began to nod and the sounds of "um hmm," "uh huh," and "you go girl" echoed throughout the room. The woman turned toward the group and after a pause rhetorically asked the group their opinion by letting out a long, drawn out, "Right?" as if it had two syllables.

Throughout the meeting, Kass had asked residents to "hold off" their questions about the assessment. Kass later explained to me that he wanted the group to have a discussion about whether spending hours or even days pouring through the health assessment and model assumptions was a good use of their time (Kass 1999). Another WABBA member spoke out and accused Kass and the consultants of being patronizing to the community by ignoring its key concern: lead poisoning.

Kass calmly explained that risk assessments rarely find a connection between an environmental exposure and health outcomes, even when such connections seem obvious to those living nearby. I observed confused looks on the faces of some WABBA members. After all, they had spent years in court arguing for the EIS and now they were being told their work may have been in vain. Another resident, in a raised voice, offered her opinion: "How could they admit to releasing lead into the air and ground and then say it will not have any 'significant' health impacts? I mean we got test results from our own kids. Let's use 'em. We didn't come this far to let 'em [the City] get away with this!"

The views of some of these WABBA members were supported by Dr. Rosen of the Albert Einstein College of Medicine. He told the group that the risk assessment models the City used were flawed and that was the reason they didn't find any health impacts from the sandblasting. "I find this to be unconscionable," Rosen said. "This whole chain of events indicates to me that the City has already disregarded the health and future growth potential of thousands of kids, who may be impacted severely and negatively by high lead exposure."

While most of the consultants assisting WABBA agreed that the lead-exposure models were "junk science," Rosen was the only professional adamant about challenging the models. He stated: "The City is doing magic tricks with the risk assessment and sweeping under the rug the real possibility that this work will result in elevated blood-lead in neighborhood children." Kass agreed that the health assessment was suspect but suggested that the best way for the group to protect children from lead poisoning might be to focus on aspects of the EIS where they could achieve "tangible gains," such as outlining a monitoring and oversight protocol with community input (Kass 1999).

As the professionals debated, WABBA seemed to splinter. A contingent of community members wanted to challenge the City's assessment by exploring the details of the model, following Rosen's advice. They insisted that tackling the model was the best thing to do because, "even if we get better monitoring procedures, we can't trust them to follow 'em anyway." This group was intent on challenging the models on the grounds that they did not use actual blood-lead levels and soil measurements from the community. Another group within WABBA argued that the risk assessment, no matter how much tweaking was done, never would prove that the lead paint released from the sandblasting contributed to elevated blood-lead levels in the community. This group wanted to work on recommendations for new community-monitoring and oversight protocols.

The first group argued loudly that WABBA had fought for the EIS and risk assessment, and they had even received financial resources from the City to critique the process, so they had an obligation to all residents to ensure the project and the assessment were as good as they could be. Ignoring the lead-poisoning issue now, many suggested, would disappoint the community. The Latina who had challenged Kass's advice later recalled the exchange with me:

There was no way we was letting the City get away with such a bogus assessment, and it seemed like some of our consultants didn't realize the situation poor people and black folks are facing. We are the ones being poisoned. It was easy for those "guys" to suggest we focus on something else. As Dr. Rosen and other experts suggested to us, if they even used actual blood-lead measurements from neighborhood kids, instead of estimates from citywide data, the risk assessment would have shown the elevated risk. We needed to change the assessment to show the City what we already knew; that their sandblasting was poisoning us.

Accusations were exchanged and some members of the coalition suggested that Kass be removed from the consulting team immediately.
Another woman stood up and shouted: " 'Y'all gotta listen to us; we
don't never get anything made for us right! Don't never get asked. . . . ' "
The woman was pumping the air with her outstretched fingers and moving her head from side to side across her shoulders for emphasis, her
body saying as much as her mouth. Because the woman was (literally)
standing tall in a sit-down meeting, and because her body language
underlined her strong feelings about the issues at hand, Kass acquiesced
to WABBA's desires. Kass later recalled, reflecting on the tense moments
at the meeting:

Some of us [public-health professionals] already had experience with risk models
around lead paint and thought the DOT models would never "prove" that the
blasting work contributed to elevated blood-lead. After all, it was never designed
as a "risk assessment," but what they called a "public health assessment."
Exactly what that meant, I'm not sure. Nonetheless, we gave the community our
honest opinion that the assessment was designed from the outset to not address
their concerns and that there was little use trying to develop a "better model."
We recommended they not waste their time picking apart the model and instead
focus on improved monitoring, oversight, alternative technologies, soil remediation—stuff that might represent tangible improvements in health, air quality,
community control, etc. The most vocal members of the group took our sugges-
tions as evidence that we were in cahoots with the City and not "on their side."
(Kass 1999)

The WABBA leadership decided to forge ahead and critique the model.
The primary concern of the community was that the model did not use
actual blood-lead samples taken specifically from affected residents
around the bridge. Instead of using local measurements, the model estimated blood-lead "baselines" by using citywide DOH lead-screening
data and developed an average "blood-lead level" based on these data.
Children's blood-lead concentrations were information community residents felt especially familiar with, since they had spent months worried
about their children's safety after the sandblasting incident. Others noted
that the City's data were especially inaccurate for their community,
because people without health insurance, like many in G/W, were less
likely to have had their children's blood tested for lead and therefore
would not be included in the City's database. Kass recalled how the
group grappled with the data inputs of the assessment:

They wanted the EIS to use real measurements taken from Williamsburg children living around the bridge. This made common-sense. Dr. Rosen was arguing that without the community specific data, the models made no sense. Even though I didn't agree with the approach, I suggested that it would be unlikely that the city would have enough data inputs using only community measurements. It was just too small a sample size. They needed a control group and from an epidemiology perspective, the city could easily discredit a model using so few samples. But, this suggestion only further alienated group members. (Kass 1999)

Rosen tried to direct the discussion over the model's assumptions. He encouraged the group to pursue its case against the City that the bridge work still presented a real threat to children's health, despite the claims in the EIS. He said it would be a great mistake to allow the work to go forward without convincing medical evidence that the sandblasting was safe. He called the recommendations of the EIS "cosmetic improvements." However, by this time many WABBA members had left the meeting frustrated over the group bickering. Additionally, Rosen, while a strong advocate, was not skilled at facilitating the group discussion. As a result, the group was unable to agree on specific recommendations for the EIS to address either the models or the monitoring procedures. Frustrated himself, Rosen gave up and decided to submit his own written comments without the endorsement of WABBA.

In the final EIS, the City agreed to encapsulate the bridge work with tarps and vacuum equipment, and the monitoring procedures were almost identical to those proposed by the mayoral task force years earlier. The community did not get independent monitors or a role in monitoring compliance, nor did the community convince the City to perform additional testing of children's blood or neighborhood soils. In fact, since the EIS claimed that there were no significant increases in soil-lead concentrations around the Williamsburg Bridge, they concluded that no additional soil remediation should be performed (DOT 1998, S-40). The City did agree to print brochures notifying the community of sandblasting work and distribute these 30 days in advance of work when possible. The sandblasting work began again in August 1999 (Liff 1999).

Making Sense of the Community Meeting

The WABBA meetings revealed the trouble community members can have articulating their local knowledge, even to sympathetic professional advisors, and how power imbalances influence this discourse. The WABBA members were unable to translate their attitudes and experiences into what could be regarded as local knowledge. This case differs significantly from, for example, the situation in chapter 3, where professionals recognized and acknowledged that if there really were anglers fishing from the river, this ought be part of the assessment. In this case, community residents were not able to get across to their own consultant why their local knowledge was important.

The WABBA members' fight with their own consultant was primarily about epistemology. The community members were trying to ask their consultants how the City's lead model, which was imported from outside the community and used data from people outside the neighborhood, could possibly be right for *their* community. The WABBA members were frustrated that the lead models didn't reflect their lived experience, and the EIS showed no sign of their years of struggle with lead poisoning. For instance, when one resident asked how a model that: "didn't take my blood, soil from my neighborhood, or show any signs of linking up with my experience that this community is polluted, be trusted?" this was an epistemological point about the nature of credible evidence. Yet, the community was not making this claim in epistemological terms—by doing such things as challenging the level of statistical analysis or sampling methods used by the city in the EIS. Thus, the meeting reveals some of the challenges community members face when attempting to make their knowledge be taken seriously and how dialogue can break down when residents make claims that are not couched in epistemological language—even when expressed to sympathetic professional advisors.

The consultants' reaction to the community members also can be understood in epistemological terms. For instance, when Kass told the group that using actual residents' blood-lead measurements would be problematic from a public-health-science standpoint because the sample size would be too small, he failed to address the crux of residents' concerns: that they did not see their experiences reflected in the City's health study. In other words, Kass did not address directly the group's primary concern about the lead model and instead shifted into a deficit model of public understanding by trying to educate residents about why their suggestion (i.e., taking samples of residents' blood for the model) would not be scientifically acceptable. Kass's reaction immediately was taken as patronizing by some members of the group, particularly when he continued to insist that WABBA should not address the model directly but instead ask for more and better monitoring. Some WABBA members were surprised that its own consultant would challenge its proposed method. The consultant's reaction also left WABBA frustrated that the health assessment would not do justice to their long-standing claims of harm. The community frustration eventually contributed to a lack of trust in their intermediaries and an end to the dialogue.

The tension at the WABBA community meeting is an example of what can happen when both community members and professional consultants sidestep the question of whose knowledge should count in community-health assessments. Local knowledge is hard to identify in this case because community members fail make their experiences and stories "fit" into categories predefined by professionals. The sympathetic professionals such as Rosen, who might have helped WABBA deconstruct the lead models failed to act as bridge-building intermediaries to help this translation occur.

The main communication challenge that surfaced in the WABBA meeting was that the professionals and the community each had different scripts they brought with them to the meeting—some visible and some hidden (Scott 1990). Scripts often include norms, values, and expectations for appropriate behavior, what constitutes emphasis versus threat, and so on, in communicative settings. They also include codes groups use, both verbal and nonverbal, that are also part of the communication process (Goffman 1959, 1971). When professionals and other actors in a social setting share life stage, ethnicity, class, and other social traits, the chance for code confusion and mistaken intentions are reduced: codes and scripts largely coincide in homogeneous settings.

However, in community planning, which most often still is conducted *by* white, middle-class professionals *in* ethnically diverse, low-income settings, common communication conventions hardly can be assumed. The same is true, of course, when planners must talk "up" to decision makers who rely on unfamiliar codes or scripts. Code confusion can lead to unwarranted and unproductive assumptions about what local people know, understand, and can learn. Such inferences may confirm the worst fears of residents about the real intentions of experts and/or the institutions that typically retain them.

Planners who are able to "code switch"—to make themselves understood in different settings—bring undeniable advantages to these encounters, but all planners can learn to observe and appreciate these aspects of communication and, armed with a knowledge of the diversity of scripts and codes, to reduce code confusion. The challenge is that professionals rarely have to "go street" in their communication settings, or switch from standard American English to a particular group's preferred informal style (Anderson 1999). However, for many people of color, this is a survival skill that enables them to effectively communicate and function in two or more social worlds or "speech communities" (Smitherman 2000). Smitherman (2000) points out that people of color in the United States historically have been forced to be more adept at this skill than other groups and the ability to code switch, or lack thereof, may explain some of the communication challenges between professionals and community members in this case.

Yet, while understanding code switching is important, it reflects only what is happening on the surface of a speech situation. Codes and scripts can be used deliberately to mask power issues. By limiting discourse to conventions of disciplinary science, professionals can perpetuate power imbalances that negate the knowledge of poor people. When street scientists say things like: "You can't be creating reliable, trustworthy, or credible evidence about me if you don't actually look at what I, for many years, have known to be a characteristic about my community," they are making an important point about both the nature of credible scientific evidence and who has the power to decide whose evidence will count in analyses.

Professional Uptake of Local Lead-Poisoning Knowledge

This episode revealed the long struggle residents endured just to be heard by professionals, and the communication challenges they encountered once they got an opportunity to consult with professionals. In the end, the WABBA coalition largely failed to influence the City that lead paint from the bridge was causing a health and environmental hazard for neighborhood residents. Yet, residents were able to influence professional decision makers to change practice (e.g., establishing the mayoral task force and creating the EIS). How community members accomplished this offers further lessons about what makes *street science* influential with professionals.

Perhaps most importantly in this case, residents successfully mobilized a coalition that included concerned community members and groups from outside the community sympathetic to their concerns. The coalition proved instrumental for gaining the attention of the media, politicians, and other professionals and for sustaining the legal effort challenging the bridge sandblasting. Without WABBA, the judge likely would not have ordered the City to pay for experts of the community's choosing. The WABBA coalition also reached beyond the borders of the neighborhood, linking the concerns of Williamsburg residents with those on the Manhattan side of the bridge and community groups across the city that might one day be impacted by bridge-paint sandblasting. WABBA also "hitched onto" the strength of a city, state, and national effort to end childhood lead poisoning. While this coalition primarily was concerned with improving lead-abatement laws and enforcement in low-income neighborhoods, WABBA successfully linked their cause with the childhood-lead-poisoning concerns more generally to take advantage of the popular attention the lead-paint-abatement advocacy had generated around the issue.

As a result of this linkage, WABBA gained significant influence with local politicians, the media, and many scientific professionals early on in the controversy. The City agreed to soil remediation, street sweeping, and the blood-lead screening program and also created the task force, all because WABBA organized and made the Williamsburg Bridge sandblasting a public issue. Admittedly, these City's responses were low-cost responses. The street cleaning and selective soil remediation were highly visible projects but had minimal environmental and health impact. The responses also were used by the City to justify their resumption of bridge sandblasting while the mitigation and studies continued. The community's knowledge and organizing efforts did not help them achieve their other goals: stopping the sandblasting, convincing the City to conduct a neighborhood blood-lead study, instituting a health-improvement program, and widespread soil remediation. The community was unable to get the City even to admit that the sandblasting might have caused dangerous lead exposures in the community and was cause for public-health intervention.

Even when backed by a mobilized coalition and successful lawsuits, *street science* will always have to grapple with entering and gaining standing within the powerful discourse of disciplinary science. As street scientists focus on gathering credible information, their efforts may be stymied—even when enlisting sympathetic professionals—if they simultaneously do not develop strategies to manage communication challenges. The final case study of *street science*, in the next chapter, highlights the opportunities and challenges for the nonverbal communication of *street science* through mapmaking.

6
The Mapping of Local Knowledge

Tell me, I forget.
Show me, I remember.
Involve me, I understand.
—Anonymous

Community scientists often map what they know about environmental health in order to communicate to both local people and professionals. Maps ranging from cartoon sketches by young people to sophisticated GIS images can powerfully display and communicate *street science*. Maps may not influence professionals, though, even when community knowledge is joined with advanced technologies such as GIS. Maps, as a medium for communicating *street science* about community environmental health problems, are crucial tools for community members. But like other modes of communication, maps can distort as much as they can reveal.

The Toxic Avengers

The Toxic Avengers was founded in 1988 by a group of high school students who organized themselves to raise community awareness about environmental pollution. The name came from a comic book of the same name, whose characters were crusaders against toxic waste.[44] The students were from the El Puente Academy high school and the community organization's program on community health, youth service, and leadership. What began as a science-class project turned into an organization that raised environmental awareness in the community and helped galvanize a community coalition that would be instrumental for taking action against neighborhood environmental hazards.

The young people who formed the Toxic Avengers were part of a science class that was doing a unit on understanding the neighborhood environment. The class researched local hazards by gathering readily available information from local, state, and federal environmental agencies on the environmental performance of facilities in the community. The students also searched through newspaper archives to find references to environmental pollution in their neighborhood. They discovered, for example, that the Radiac Corporation—a storage and transfer facility for toxic, flammable, and low-level-radioactive waste located in the neighborhood—was the only facility of its kind in the entire city.

The class instructors, with the help of local environmental activists and agency professionals, organized environmental "tours" of the neighborhood. Environmental professionals and activists often led these "toxic tours" in which students visited the local sewage-treatment plant, natural-gas tank farm, waste-transfer station, scrap-metal recycling facility, Superfund site, depot for sanitation trucks, and other locally noxious industries. Students also identified the "green" spaces in the neighborhood. On the tours, the gravity of each environmental insult often was felt immediately because of fumes, odors, or noise levels. While on the tours, students took photos and recorded their observations, feelings, and perceptions about each site.

The students returned to the classroom and were tasked with developing a "community-risk map." Community-risk mapping is a process adapted from the practices of labor organizers, often in farming and other industries, where potential health and safety risks exist in the workplace (Hesperian Foundation 1998; Mujica 1992; Smith, Barret, and Box et al. 2000). In workplace-risk mapping, workers identify and categorize risks they face then plot them on maps of their work environments. Workers are encouraged to use symbols and other nontraditional mapping devices to display the locations of areas or tasks in the workplace where they have experienced or perceived dangerous or noxious conditions (Mujica 1992). Community-risk mapping emulates the workplace mapping process and generally involves a group brainstorming session to list hazards, code and symbolize these hazards, and then map them on large poster-board. The process, also analogous with community "visioning" sessions commonly used for planning purposes, can be particularly effective when used in communities where residents may be uncomfortable with public speaking or technical information, are not fluent in English, and seek a means for creatively expressing how they perceive their neighborhood (Aberley 1993; Ames 1998).

The Toxic Avengers used what they learned in science class to develop a map of the community for the explicit purpose of organizing residents. After learning that an upcoming public hearing would be reviewing the operating permit of the Radiac waste storage and transfer facility, the students decided to use their map of the neighborhood to draw attention to the poorly maintained and, in their eyes, dangerous facility. The Avengers came up with a map that became affectionately known as the Skulls map (figure 6.1). The map was turned into a

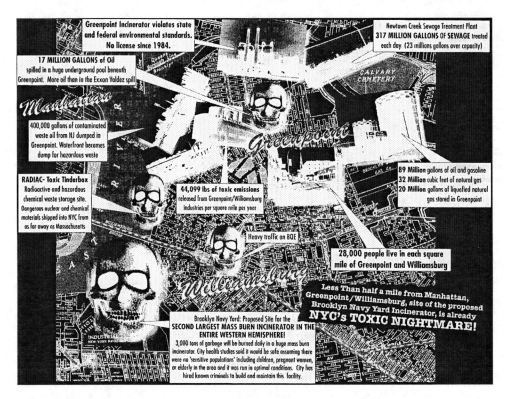

Figure 6.1.
Toxic Avengers skulls map. Source: El Puente Toxic Avengers.

poster and used to publicize the Radiac hearing throughout the neighborhood. The risk-mapping process created more than a new image of the community. The process itself helped build a new network of young activists, created a new organization for young people to express their knowledge, and helped galvanize other community members to consider the environmental-health challenges in front of them.

What Maps Do

Maps perform at least three political functions in relation to knowledge. First, maps always *aggregate and select data* and how they do this can lead to enormous differences in interpretive outcomes. Second, maps are *identity forming* devices since the symbols used to visually present information give "life" and persuasiveness to certain representations. Third, maps are always *boundary makers* by including some information and excluding others.

Aggregation

How maps aggregate information for visual presentation may lead to enormous differences in interpretive outcomes. The maps and images that are used as standard ways of seeing a problem tell us whose vision matters, what should be rendered visible, and what should be made invisible. Maps are also always made for certain purposes, such as to convince an audience of a certain point of view, and they provide rules for real-world decisions. A particular map "wins" or becomes the dominant image of the day by resonating with those in political power (Scott 1998). For example, *National Geographic* often is cited for generating maps during the Cold War with an explicitly Western perspective; the Soviet Union was portrayed as a large (and presumably dangerous) land mass compared to Europe and the United States. Similarly, maps of the world often have portrayed Africa as smaller and less prominent (and thus less important) compared to Europe and North America (Monmonier 1996).

Yet, the power of maps for (mis)representing reality remains a contentious subject in planning, science, and policymaking. Harley (1989) notes that maps represent hypothetical generalizations and are always, to some degree, inaccurate. They model a reality known to be more complex than any map can portray. Yet, at the same time, maps exert a compelling persuasiveness; they are designed to look real—particularly to those beyond the mapmaking community (Monmonier 1996).

Boundary Making

Mapmaking also can be understood as a scientific process, where some information is selected and others excluded in order to make the project legible (Lynch and Woolgar 1990). For example, Gieryn (1995) notes how mapmaking acts as a powerful metaphor for understanding the production of scientific knowledge itself. Science often is portrayed as an "empty map" that becomes filled in by certain groups or institutions in order to have influence over a particular audience. The "mapmaking" of science is the decision to include and exclude certain information, and thereby to create boundaries around what counts as science. In other words mapping, like science, always shows a limited representation of a complex reality and generates provisional, contextual, and always amendable information (Gieryn 1995, 406).

Yet, the production of visual images can extend the influence of science, often taking on a life of its own. For example, Latour (1988) introduces the idea of the "immutable mobile," which is an image such as a map that is a fixed display of information and is used in different times and contexts to represent ideas or facts. One common example is the picture of the earth suspended in space, which has come to represent such things as environmentalism, holism, peace, and a number of other things. The meaning of the image, how it was produced, and by whom often is taken for granted or even ignored when it is used.

Ultimately, the legitimacy and credibility of a map is judged by what the cartographers choose to include in the physical rendering and the trustworthiness of the cartographers themselves. By creating boundaries around what is and is not important to see, maps can encourage viewers to "see like the state" or suggest some other imagined vision (Anderson 1991; Scott 1998). As Harley notes; mapmaking is a political process that deserves a critical analysis:

All maps strive to frame their message in the context of an audience. All maps state an argument about the world and they are propositional in nature. All maps employ the common devices of rhetoric such as invocations of authority and appeals to a potential readership through the use of colors, decoration, typography, dedications, and written justifications of their method. Rhetoric may be concealed, but it is always present, for there is no description without performance. (Harley 1989, 11)

Thus, the mapmaking "performance" should be recognized as a political process that can reveal much about the society within which the image is created.

Identity Formation

Ultimately, while maps are models of reality, they also shape that reality. In environmental planning, maps often reflect the views of scientists and policy makers about what knowledge and whose perspectives are authoritative, whether one or a plurality of plausible interpretations are legitimate, and at what scale a problem ought to be addressed (i.e., local, state, federal). For example, land-use maps are often de facto "base maps" used to describe the attributes of a place, implicitly suggesting that making physical changes to the land-use of a place is the principal means to address local issues (Hayden 1995). Peter Hall (1994) argues that the widespread institutional acceptance of land use mapping has helped perpetuate the "functionalist" view of city planning as the dominant paradigm in the field. In the functionalist view, planning is defined by how professionals label, demarcate, and separate land uses into zones and classify these areas by their function. In this case, mapping and particular types of standardized maps, have defined an entire field.

One of the most common tools used to model reality in urban planning today is the geographic information system (GIS). The GIS technology is a means of integrating spatial and nonspatial information into a single computer system for analysis and graphical display. The technology allows users to input vast amounts of information, perform statistical spatial analyses, and generate images of data analyses that extend the vision of the modern geographer. However, the reliance on computer-generated maps has been criticized for raising obstacles for public participation in and understanding of the mapping process. For instance, lay publics, especially those from disadvantaged groups, may have limited knowledge of and access to computers. Since the assumptions underlying computer-produced maps are buried within the computer application itself, GIS may further hinder lay understanding of the mapping process. Yet, at the same time, the increased availability of computing power also might lead to the democratization (or at least accountability) of map-making, precisely because citizen groups may be able to offer their own computer-generated maps.

The "GIS revolution" in planning has perpetuated an almost unfettered trust by both users and consumers of planning information in quantitative data as the most legitimate information for generating accurate spatial analyses, making maps, and ultimately characterizing places. Another emerging implication is that the technology is beginning to frame social problems as spatial research questions. In a note of irony and precaution, Monmonier (1996) reveals that the errors, inaccuracies, and imprecision inherent in GIS devolve from one of the technology's greatest strengths: the ability to collate and cross-reference many types of data and discrete data sets by location, called "geo-coding," in a single system. As new data sets are imported, the GIS also can inherit its errors and combine these with errors already in the system. Users of GIS must concern themselves as much with "cleaning" disparate data sets to match one another as with devising strategies to visually display the data.

As professionals increasingly rely on GIS in their work, some are making efforts to incorporate public stakeholders, especially community members, into the spatial mapmaking process (Aberley 1993). Efforts at public participation in GIS often include processes to incorporate local knowledge into data sets (Craig and Elwood 1998; Robbins 2003). As community members increasingly become both producers and consumers of GIS, planning processes and participants will continue to be shaped by this and other professional mapping technologies.

Maps as Organizers of Attention

The Toxic Avengers' Skulls map (figure 6.1) describes the neighborhood as "NYC's toxic nightmare." It shows skulls describing numerous local hazards and uses both graphic visuals and text. The background, or base map, is a photocopied tax-surveyor map made to look like an X-ray, enhancing the sense of urgency that pollution is compromising personal health. Photographs of industrial facilities used to identify the locations of particular polluters personalize the map for local residents since most would recognize the facilities. However, the pictures were slightly "whited out" to look almost ghostly.

The Toxic Avengers brought the map to Luis Garden-Acosta, El Puente's founder and executive director, in an effort to encourage him to personally invite the neighborhood's Hasidic Jewish population to the Radiac hearing. After seeing the map, Acosta was convinced that all the community's ethnic groups would need to work together to improve environmental conditions (Hevesi 1994). According to Garden-Acosta:

It was nothing but confrontation [with the Hasidim] before young people from the Toxic Avengers came to me and said, "Isn't it time to ask the Hasidim to join forces with us in reclaiming our environment?" It was their request and their graphic map gave me the "ah ha" that we all breathe the same air. (quoted in Hevesi 1994)

Acosta sent an invitation to Rabbi David Niederman, executive director of the UJO of Williamsburg, to come to a planning meeting for the Radiac event. Niederman agreed to meet with El Puente and bring other Hasidim with him after El Puente agreed to hire police to guarantee their security. As Garden-Acosta recounts those events in May 1991:

It was a historic moment when a Hasidic rabbi, a leader of the Satmar, walked through the doors of El Puente. We were planning a march to a hearing on Radiac emergency procedures, and Rabbi Niederman volunteered to help lead that march through Latino streets. I can't describe what a change that meant. It was a clear act of courage on the part of David Niederman. (quoted in Hevesi 1994)

The multiethnic march raised interest in the issues, and over 200 people attended the hearing. The success of the event encouraged the two groups to organize an "environmental town meeting" to raise awareness about local hazards and specifically to educate residents about a proposed municipal waste incinerator in the Brooklyn Navy Yard. According to Niederman, the meeting was necessary because no group alone could confront the multiple environmental threats the community faced: "We were facing the incinerator, lead poisoning, garbage transfer stations, chemicals from abandoned factories around here, sandblasting from the bridge and Radiac. We had to come together" (quoted in Hevesi 1994).

The incinerator proposal galvanized the community, which saw the project as treating their homes as the dumping ground for unwanted garbage. The incinerator was supposed to be the most cost-effective way for the City to dispose of municipal solid waste. In the 1980s, after closing all but one landfill and most of its incinerators, New York City feared a garbage-disposal crisis. The possibility of a crisis made headlines in 1987 when a garbage barge called the "Mobro," carrying 32,206 tons of NY refuse, left Islip on a six-month journey in search of a place to unload. The barge, turned away by several states and three countries, eventually returned to New York; most of its garbage was burned at the Southwest Brooklyn incinerator (Miller 2000). Soon thereafter, the City devised a comprehensive solid-waste management plan that would close the 22 City-operated incinerators and the over 1,200 private apartment-building incinerators. In order to handle its waste, the City planned to build eight new incinerators and the Williamsburg facility was planned as the first and largest (Miller 2000).

The Brooklyn Navy Yard incinerator was proposed as a "state of the art" facility that could burn nearly one-third of the city's daily municipal waste (approximately 3,000 tons per day at the time of the proposal) and was supposed to ease the burden on the only operating landfill site in the city, Fresh Kills on Staten Island (Waldman 1997). At the time, the largest incinerator in the city was burning 550 tons per day. Neighborhood residents, along with city, state, and national environmental groups sued the City to stop the proposed project based on the expected increased truck traffic and unsafe air emissions (Liff 1992; Sullivan 1995). Barry Commoner, who emerged as a vocal opponent of the project, claimed that dioxins from the incinerator would poison local residents (Commoner 1992, 109–119).

The town meeting brought together community leaders representing different issues and ethnic groups to speak about hazards in the community and the need to organize together to stop the incinerator. According to Elizabeth Colon, executive officer of the Brooklyn Navy Yard corporation, the meting was as much about the future direction of community development, particularly concerns over the changing economic realities in the neighborhood, including "unemployment and a deteriorating economic base," as about environmental issues (Hevesi 1994). Residents also feared that if the City was allowed to build an incinerator on the property of one obsolete industrial site, a similar fate would await the hundreds of other decaying and abandoned industrial properties scattered around the neighborhood.

The Toxic Avengers helped develop another map of the community. The "Our Town" map (figure 6.2) was intended to show that the community was under multiple environmental stressors, not just the proposed incinerator. Like the Skulls map, the Our Town map used graphic displays of death and danger to portray the neighborhood. Skulls and crossbones were used to label toxic storage sites, a large nuclear symbol identified the Radiac facility, and black smoke was shown coming from stacks to identify the proposed incinerator sites around the community. The Our Town map also was filled with descriptive information about the amount of pollution emitted from local facilities.

Over 1,200 residents attended the environmental town meeting, which ended with a commitment from leaders of the Latino, Hasidic, African-American, and Polish communities to form the Community Alliance for the Environment (Greider 1993).[45] The first action CAFE planned was a multiethnic march over the Williamsburg Bridge during rush hour to protest the proposed incinerator (Hevesi 1994).[46] The Toxic Avengers' map helped educate and organize the new multiethnic environmental coalition. The 1992 march has been credited as one of the key turning points that eventually convinced the City to mothball the incinerator proposal (Sullivan 1995).

Both the Skulls and Our Town maps reveal the creativity and awareness young people can bring to an environmental issue. They suggest that, as Mumford noted, the planning process often begins "with a dynamic emotional urge, springing out of a sense of frustration on one hand and a renewed vision of life on the other" (1938, 359). The maps acted as powerful representations of a "dying neighborhood" inundated with hazards. On each map, almost no space was left for viewers to see what else was in the neighborhood besides the polluting facilities. The maps help "pattern attention selectively," or reveal what some residents' value. They publicly express allegiances and prepared residents "to recognize new issues and attend creatively and responsively to particular struggles at hand" (Forester 1999, 139). The maps accomplished their mission of organizing and galvanizing an important multiethnic environmental coalition in the neighborhood.

Students were able to combine local knowledge and professional data into powerful visual information. Visualizing local knowledge, whether

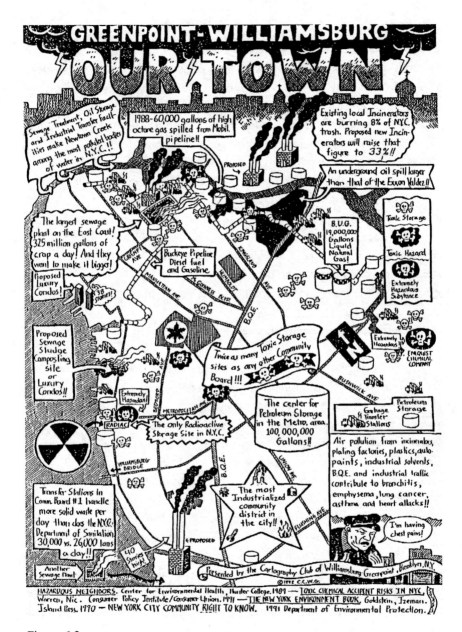

Figure 6.2.
"Our Town" community map. Source: Cartography Club of Williamsburg/
Greenpoint.

through community maps, murals, or theater, allows local people to express what they know, share it with other community members in a way that is understandable for all, focus discussion, and propose options for action. As tools for educating community members, sharing experiences, and mobilizing action, maps can be as or more important than local knowledge as text, particularly in communities with disparate levels of formal education, common language, symbols, and traditions. But while the student maps showed that mapping local knowledge can be important for influencing people *within* the community, it is less useful for relating to outside professionals.

The student maps gave "voice" to those previously silent about environmental hazards and showed how residents perceived local pollution and its impacts on different groups within the neighborhood. And while the maps did not help extend professional science, they stimulated community interest in developing other visual portraits of neighborhood pollution.

Contested Images: Community and Professional Maps

The student maps were low-tech images that contained a lot of detail but were cartoonlike. Community groups realized during the incinerator battle that they would have to start generating maps to compete with technical experts in order to make their point of cumulative environmental impacts in the neighborhood (Swanston 1999). Soon after CAFE formed, the Watchperson Project was created. Part of the Watchperson Project's charter included developing GIS and making it accessible for community members (ICLEI 1993; Sweeney et al. 1994). Beginning in 1993, the Watchperson Project partnered with Hunter College to gather electronic data to enter into a community-based GIS. A key goal for the community was to use the GIS for analyzing the proximity of polluters to residents and to develop sophisticated and "official looking" maps (Hanhardt 1999). The Watchperson Project initially used GIS to produce maps displaying the relationship between hazards and residents, schools, and other sensitive receptors. One of the first published maps displayed the proximity of the Radiac facility, an electroplater, and a sugar factory to a school, day care center, and neighborhood playground (figure 6.3). The community first used the GIS to challenge a City-backed project during a

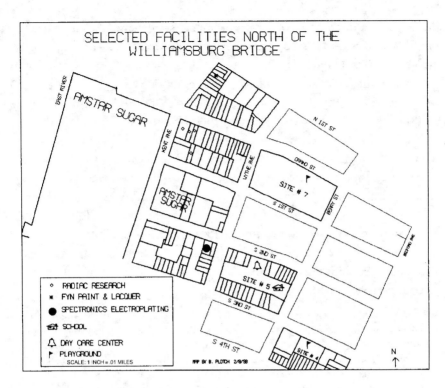

Figure 6.3.
GIS map depicting selected facilities north of the Williamsburg Bridge. Source:
Watchperson Project.

public hearing over the permitting of a controversial waste-transfer station in the neighborhood.

In April 1998, the city Department of Sanitation (DOS) and the state
Department of Environmental Conservation (DEC) approved the siting of
the largest waste-transfer station in the city's history.[47] The transfer station, which was permitted to process up to 5,000 tons of waste per day on
the Kent Avenue site known as Eastern District Terminal, would be operated by the USA Waste Services Corporation (Saltonstall 1998).[48] The
60,000-square-foot facility was approved by the DOS and DEC without
an assessment of potential environmental, traffic, and public health
impacts. The agencies granted the facility a "Neg Dec," declaring that the
facility posed no potential significant impact on the community. A coalition of community organizations sued the state claiming that the size of

the facility required an environmental impact statement.[49] A public hearing, the required final step in the permitting process, was held in April after the facility's approval.

Representatives from a number of community groups testified against the proposed facility. From restaurant owners, who said the noise, dust, and smell of the facility would destroy their business, to community leaders such as Rabbi Niederman, who claimed that the trucks and pollution would put all community residents at risk. The testimonials of over 200 residents occupied almost the entire hearing and carried the proceeding well past midnight.[50] An administrative law judge presided over the hearing. Samara Swanston, presented a series of maps showing the areas in the community that would be impacted, such as those along truck routes. The maps also showed the number of existing waste-transfer stations and their proximity to low-income and minority-group populations. According to Swanston:

We tried to make the case that not only was this mammoth facility going to hurt business, it was also part of a pattern of environmental injustice in the neighborhood. When community folks start talking about environmental justice, regulators tend to cringe, and that is what the DEC did. But, the ALJ [administrative law judge] was more open. I think he hadn't really heard of the issue before. When we put up the map of the cumulative hazards and I asked him if he'd want his kids to live here, he kind of did a double take. (Swanston 1999)

The cumulative hazard map showed the truck routes, the locations of the neighborhood's transfer stations, school and park properties, and sites where toxins were used and released (figure 6.4). The map also plotted the locations where elevated lead levels were found in neighborhood children, an oil plume underneath the neighborhood, and the sewage treatment plant. According to Heather Roslund, an activist with Neighbors Against Garbage (NAG), the map was significant because:

It gave us legitimacy. We not only gave our testimony, but we showed them [DEC and DOS] that we also did our homework and had technical skills. The community maps showed that we were not just about NIMBY, but that this was a much larger issue about environmental hazards and social justice. We showed that we were prepared and could go head-to-head with the city, state and even a big corporation like USA Waste.

The DOS countered the community's presentation with maps of their own. The DOS argued that this was a siting case and that the facilities

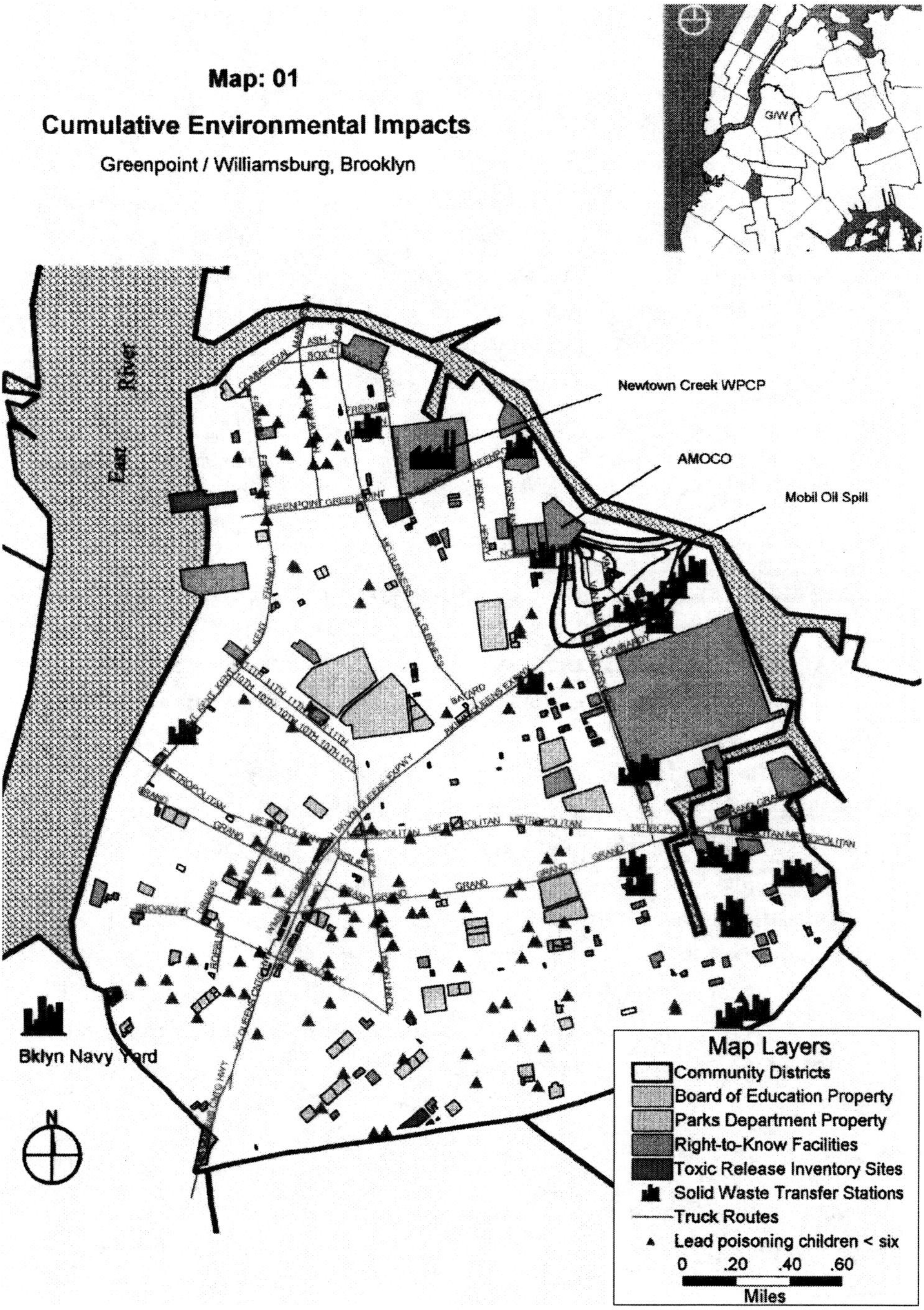
Map: 01
Cumulative Environmental Impacts
Greenpoint / Williamsburg, Brooklyn
G/W
East River
Newtown Creek WPCP
AMOCO
Mobil Oil Spill
Bklyn Navy Yard
N
Map Layers
Community Districts
Board of Education Property
Parks Department Property
Right-to-Know Facilities
Toxic Release Inventory Sites
Solid Waste Transfer Stations
Truck Routes
Lead poisoning children < six
0 .20 .40 .60
Miles

Figure 6.4.
Cumulative-environmental-impact map. Source: Watchperson Project.

were necessary to avoid a garbage-disposal crisis. The issue, according to the DOS, was about available appropriately zoned land. The City displayed a map of the neighborhood's zoning and land use. The only other environmental features on the map were truck routes and the location of existing transfer stations (figure 6.5). The City argued that the only legal location for transfer stations was in areas zoned for heavy manufacturing, labeled "M-zones," and G/W happened to have more of this land than almost any other community district in the city. According to James Doherty, sanitation commissioner at the time:

The only clustering we might see of transfer stations is because these facilities are limited to industrial areas and these tend to be concentrated in certain parts of the city. In fact, we even exempted the light-industrial, M-1 zones, which tend to be closest to residential areas. We [DOS] have no control over where these things get sited. They go where the zoning allows them to go. (quoted in Martin 1998)

The City's maps were used as a justification for the permitting of the waste-transfer station and were used to deflect concerns about injustice and whether G/W was a community already overburdened with hazards.

In the eyes of most community members, the maps were an indication of the City's refusal to acknowledge the cumulative toxic burden facing the neighborhood. The City's maps became known by residents as the "toxic donut" maps. They showed the oval-shaped community surrounded on all sides by manufacturing land uses and industrial zones, with residents living in the center of the industrial ring.

The administrative law judge overseeing the hearing ruled that the community's case was compelling and required USA Waste to provide more information to show that their facility would not have a significant environmental impact on local residents. The judge ruled that it seemed "unreasonable" for a facility of such a size not to have some impact on the community, and, in light of the background environmental conditions in the community, more information would be necessary before any permits granted (Shin 1999). In June of 1998, both the New York State Assembly and Senate passed bills (S7610/A11084), introduced by Brooklyn representatives, requiring USA Waste to perform an EIS. And, just two months after the hearing, on June 23, 1998, Governor Pataki signed the bill and announced that the State would require USA Waste to prepare the environmental assessment.[51] However, after a year of study,

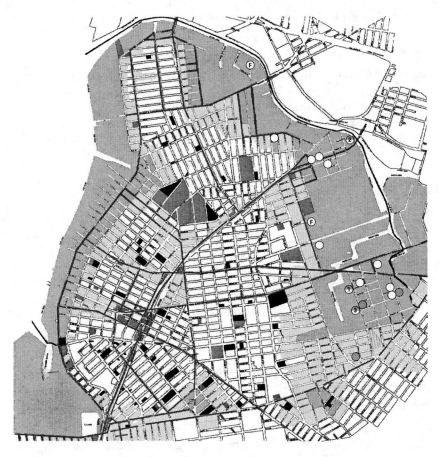

Brooklyn
Community Board 1

☐ Residential or commercial
▨ Manufacturing Zone M1
▨ Manufacturing Zone M2 & M3
■ School
▨ Park

◯ Non-putresible transfer station
⬤ Putresible transfer station
Ⓕ Fill transfer station

━ D.O.T. truck rout

Figure 6.5.
New York City zoning map and locations of transfer stations in Greenpoint/
Williamsburg. Source: New York City Department of City Planning.

the EIS concluded that there would again be "no significant impacts" from the facility but, at the urging of Congresswoman Nydia Velazquez, the White House Council on Environmental Quality and the EPA began an examination into whether G/W had been targeted for garbage-transfer stations because residents were poor and minorities (Shin 1999). According to Brad Campell, a CEQ associate director:

The problems we see here have a huge influence on policy and legislation. We were very disappointed that the City Housing, Sanitation and Environmental Protection departments are not joining us in this effort. The best chance for solutions is when we have a partnership between federal, state and local governments. (quoted in Shin 1999)

As the federal investigation went ahead, the DOS granted the waste-transfer station its permit. It wasn't until May 2000, after the NY Lawyers for the Public Interest (representing the community) convinced a Manhattan Supreme Court judge to block the permit, that the facility finally stopped operating (Liff 2000).

By combining agency data with residents' experience of hazards, the community hazard map was attempting to extend the work of professional science. The community map also tried to shift the debate from facility siting and zoning to cumulative impacts and environmental injustice. However, the City perceived the map as a threat and countered that it was "irrelevant" for siting decisions that were based on zoning. The map did help residents gain attention from the environmental justice movement, and this visibility played a significant role in getting the federal government and eventually the administrative law judge to pay attention to the community's claims. Community mapping played a key role organizing attention but ultimately only supplemented the legal arguments that influenced professional action.

Mapping Small-Source Air Polluters

As environmental justice claims continued to surface in the neighborhood,[52] community groups continued expanding the capabilities of their own GIS. The Watchperson Project used its mapping technology to influence the EPA's Cumulative Exposure Project (CEP), the same project that assessed risks from subsistence fish diets discussed in chapter 3. This time, the community mapped polluters that an EPA exposure model in the community would have overlooked.

While the relationship between air pollution and public health long has been studied (ATS 1996; Holgate et al. 1999), definitive conclusions about air pollution's effects on urban residents are limited. In addition to gaps in understanding regarding the biologic mechanisms responsible for the morbidity and mortality associated with increased air pollution, a lack of consistent ambient monitoring in urban areas has prevented scientists from capturing pollution at the local or microenvironment level. Yet, high concentrations of air pollutants are suspected of being common in many poor urban neighborhoods. The lack of microenvironment air monitoring also has prevented study of intra-urban or neighborhood differences that also might help better understand distributions of health effects associated with urban air pollutants. Additionally, combining point, area, and mobile sources to characterize pollution in microenvironments has proved difficult. Thus, dispersion models are used to estimate micro-scale urban pollution.

The CEP's first task of the air toxic exposure assessment involved gathering data inputs for the hazardous-air-pollutant (HAP) dispersion model called, Assessment System for Population Exposure Nationwide (ASPEN). The ASPEN model estimates long-term outdoor concentrations of 148 of the 188 HAPs listed in the Clean Air Act of 1970 for every census tract in the contiguous United States, based on 1990 data (totaling 60,803 census tracts) (EPA 1999a; Rosenbaum et al. 1999; Woodruff et al. 1998). ASPEN is a Gaussian dispersion model that estimates outdoor concentrations of HAPs on the basis of their emission rates, frequency of various meteorologic conditions, and the effects of atmospheric processes such as decay, secondary formation, and deposition.

The EPA planned on using the ASPEN model in G/W and adding any relevant local emission sources. However, the agency was content on basing the model on pollution data from the one NYS DEC air monitor in the neighborhood and the roughly fifty Toxic Release Inventory (TRI) sites registered with the EPA that were known to emit some hazardous air pollutants (EPA 1999a). During meetings presenting the project to the community, EPA heard from residents that their proposed methodology, particularly the census-tract aggregation and the reliance solely on state and federal data, was going to miss some potentially hazardous exposures. According to a local resident attending one of the meetings:

If you just walk around here you can see that we've got polluters mixed in with residents; some small and other large factories. To tell us that everyone in the census tract was exposed more or less the same missed the variations on the street.

More specifically, representatives from the Watchperson Project noted that the air-dispersion model was going to miss hundreds of potential polluters because they did not show up in any state or federal air-quality database. These polluters were registered, since they had to file for permits with the NYC DEP, but their emissions were not monitored. According to community members commenting on the EPA analysis, the census-tract aggregation of the ASPEN model was going to "wash out" the block-to-block pollution differences that existed in the neighborhood. The Watchperson Project noted that the air toxic model made no mention of indoor air pollution, specifically perchloroethylene ("perc"), a known carcinogen suspected of affecting residents living above dry cleaners (Swanston 2000).

In making their case to the EPA, community residents once again developed their own set of maps. The Watchperson Project used their GIS to develop maps comparing the state hazardous sites the EPA used as data inputs for the model to the DEP-regulated air polluters that the model was slated to ignore (figure 6.6). The Watchperson Project had spent over two years trying to obtain environmental information from the City, including air-permit information, environmental complaints records, and parcel-by-parcel tax information from the City's Department of Finance. The DEP data was from the Bureau of Air Resources Administration Management Information System and included permit data on over 3,000 facilities in the neighborhood that were required to file for an air-emission permit but were not regulated, such as apartment-building boilers, auto-body paint shops, and printers. The Department of Finance data set included details about the history of every land parcel in the neighborhood for tax assessment purposes, and included information such as building type, property value, fire department inspections, and property owner. After a lengthy battle with the City, including numerous Freedom of Information Act requests, the community group obtained the electronic data (Swanston 1999). The Watchperson Project was the only community organization in the City that obtained these disparate data sets and, since these data were not housed at any one agency, no agency had compiled this information into one computer system capable of graphically displaying the information (Hanhardt 1999). With the help of computer specialists from Hunter College, the group began manipulating the data in their own GIS.

The Watchperson Project's map showing the block-by-block variation of air polluters was aimed at convincing the EPA that their model's aggregation was not fine-grained enough to accurately characterize air pollution in the neighborhood. According to Robert Lewis, director of the Watchperson's Office GIS project:

> To capture data only by census tract or block group averaged-out significant localized emissions. A data-set that aggregated by census-tract or even block would miss important distinctions between city blocks and even within one block. We had the data to show this. So we produced maps of the entire neighborhood and presented them to EPA showing just how many small-sources there are in the neighborhood and how the state and federal databases missed all these. (Lewis 2000)

The Watchperson Project mapped 15,167 distinct land parcels in the community and produced maps comparing the facilities used in the EPA model with facilities regulated by the DEP but which the dispersion model was not going to include (e.g. figure 6.6). The group found over 1,000 potentially toxic air polluters that the EPA would miss in its census-tract level assessment (Swanston 2000).

The Watchperson Project's maps were convincing to EPA scientists, but the agency struggled with how to treat the information in their dispersion model. According to one EPA scientist:

> The community maps made sense, especially after some of us had toured the neighborhood with some residents. We had a sense there were lots of small sources, but we didn't realize the full extent until we saw the community's maps. We struggled for a long time considering what to do with their data set. We tweaked the model some but we just couldn't aggregate all those sources at a block-by-block level without loosing accuracy in the dispersion model. What we did do, however, was take the area sources we could get enough data for, plot them, and model them as point sources.[53]

The community-generated map forced EPA to rethink whether its dispersion model was an accurate characterization of on-the-ground exposures, but it ultimately did not significantly alter the agency's dispersion model.

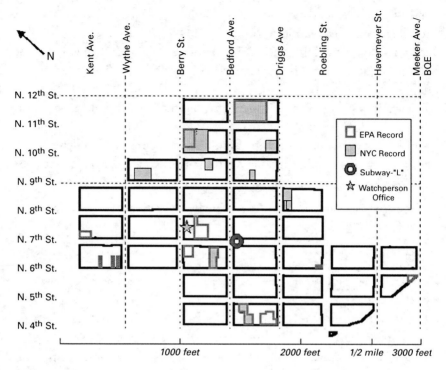

Figure 6.6.
Community-generated block-by-block map comparing EPA and DEP modeling sites. Source: Watchperson Project.

A second map produced by the Watchperson Project's GIS was also used to try to influence the EPA modelers. As part of their GIS program, the community group used volunteer high-school students to canvass the neighborhood in teams to follow up on community complaints of air, noise, and odor pollution registered by residents with the DEP. The community group plotted the location of the complaints on GIS-generated maps and students "investigated" the areas near the complaints to look for any obvious sources of pollution that might need attention. One finding from the student's "street survey" was that a large number of complaints were coming from residents living in buildings with dry cleaning establishments (Swanston 2000).

After learning about the findings of the student canvass, the Watchperson Project organized a special project focused on documenting the location of all neighborhood dry-cleaning establishments and the specific type of buildings in which they were located. The survey found 54 dry cleaners in the neighborhood, with 23 of the 54 performing dry-cleaning in a residential building (EPA 1999a). Using the GIS and census data, the community group estimated that as many as 183 apartments and approximately 550 residents were living above dry-cleaning establishments (EPA 1999a). Again the group mapped these findings and presented them to the EPA modelers (figure 6.7).

The Watchperson Project's dry-cleaning survey raised a particular concern to EPA since a number of recent studies in New York City had found concentrations of perc inside apartments, at up to three floors above a dry cleaner in the same building, averaging 150 ppm (parts per million), with some measurements exceeding 1,000 ppm (Wallace et al. 1995; NYS DOH 1993).[54] In one study by the NYS DOH, 39 of 40 apartments above dry cleaners tested had concentrations of perc in the air exceeding the 100 ppm state guideline for noncancer effects. One measurement in this study found perc levels at 197,000 ppm. Another study by the Consumers Union found that 24 of 29 apartments above dry cleaners had four-day average concentrations of perc above the DOH guideline and 8 had average concentrations above 1,000 ppm (Wallace et al. 1995).

The EPA ASPEN model estimated the expected *outdoor* concentration of perc at less than 2 ppb (part per billion), with a maximum-modeled census-tract outdoor concentration of 39 ppb (EPA 1999a). According to Fred Talcott, Project Director of the CEP at EPA:

The average concentration found in apartments above dry cleaning establishments was on the order of 1,000 times higher than the outdoor concentration of "perc" as predicted by the ASPEN model in G/W. That to me is an illustration of a micro-level problem that would be completely obscured if you only looked at daily walking around concentration. Without the community group data set, we would have missed this. (Talcott 1999)

EPA considered performing a separate assessment for this subpopulation, but eventually decided to document the findings only in the CEP report (EPA 1999a, 6–24).

These two examples of community mapping reveal that local knowledge can bring important insights to sophisticated technological assessments. The community GIS organized information that no other agency

LOCATION OF DRY CLEANERS IN GREENPOINT/WILLIAMSBURG

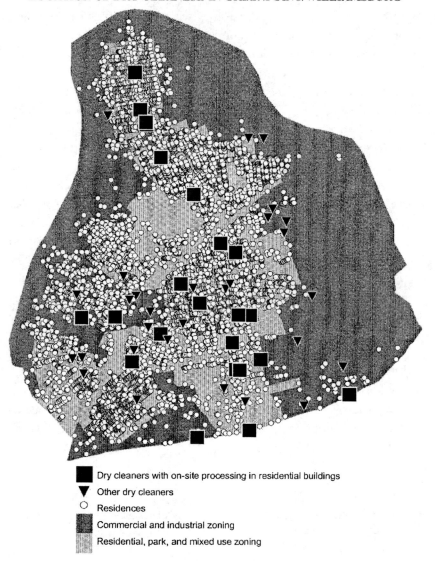

Dry cleaners with on-site processing in residential buildings

▼ Other dry cleaners

○ Residences

Commercial and industrial zoning

Residential, park, and mixed use zoning

Figure 6.7.
Community plots of neighborhood dry cleaners. Source: US EPA 1999a, chapter 6, p. 23.

had compiled and then mapped these data to reveal what daily experience already told most residents: that pollution exposures differ from block-to-block and even along the same block. The community group also combined their computer-mapping capabilities with a student survey to find a hazard unanticipated by the EPA: potential toxic exposures from dry cleaners in residential buildings. In both instances, the community-mapping technology helped validate what residents already were experiencing (e.g., following up on air and odor complaints) and helped bring this knowledge to the attention of the EPA. While the community maps failed in the end to significantly alter the EPA air-dispersion model, the maps did challenge the EPA to address new questions, new sources of data, new exposures, and new groups claiming access to the assessment process—all of which had a significant impact on the way professionals viewed their role, if not their final decisions.

How Community Maps Influence Professionals

Maps are an important tool for organizing and making publicly visible the *street science* performed in communities. The mapping of local knowledge in G/W ranged from student drawings on photocopied street maps to sophisticated computer-generated GIS outputs. In each instance, maps were used as counter expertise, opposing a noxious facility or challenging professional assumptions about how to assess the neighborhood's environment. In each case, residents eventually changed the way professionals viewed the environmental issue at stake, although the extent to which the community maps were responsible for these changes was mixed.

The Toxic Avenger's maps did not directly influence professionals but, by helping organize the community around environmental issues, the student maps helped build an important coalition that played a role influencing professional decisions. The community's cumulative burdens map was a key piece of a series of influential testimony that convinced the administrative law judge and other politicians to eventually demand that USA Waste perform an EIS. However, the community's hazard map was not convincing to the City, as they continued to permit the transfer station even after the federal government intervened. For the City, the issue was appropriate zoning, not cumulative environmental impacts or unfair sit-ing practices. It took successful litigation two years after the initial public hearing to convince the City to revoke the transfer station's permit. Finally, the GIS maps that the Watchperson Project offered to the EPA modelers were compelling, even mapping information that no other agency could combine, but did not significantly alter the air dispersion model.

In this case, the student maps were explicitly aimed at building a com-munity coalition, but the other maps were not. The student maps com-bined understandings from agency databases, environmental pollution information, and local experiences with pollution. However, the maps were more expressions of how a group of local people saw the conditions under which they lived and the cartoonlike use of symbols might have contributed to professionals not taking these maps seriously. The com-munity's GIS-generated maps combined electronic information that agencies and scientists were themselves using with local knowledge of problems and experiences with hazards. These *street science* maps both extended the understanding of scientists and also radically challenged professional analyses. For example, the GIS maps identified small-source air polluters that the EPA model was going to miss and helped fill gaps in the agency's modeling inputs. The cumulative environmental impacts map radically challenged the fairness of the City's transfer-station-siting practices and attempted to shift the discourse from zoning to environ-mental justice.

The influence of expert intermediaries was less significant in these episodes because visual images tend to "speak for themselves." The com-munity did use intermediaries to help them obtain some electronic data and build their GIS, however. In some ways, the GIS technology itself acted as the surrogate intermediary, since the technology was something both professionals and locals accepted as a legitimate means for display-ing environmental information. The more the street scientists were able to make their knowledge resemble professional renditions, the more pro-fessionals took their work seriously.

As these episodes reveal, community-generated maps can challenge radically the way professionals are normally prepared to address environmental health problems. When community groups reframed the waste-transfer-station issue as one about fairness and justice by using their cumulative-hazard map, the City could not respond. Even when the federal government intervened to investigate whether waste-transfer stations were being targeted for poor and minority neighborhoods, the City refused to participate in this probe. Similarly, the EPA modelers could find no easy solution to the inadequacy of the census-tract-level aggregation of their air dispersion model, or for keeping the model from missing hundreds of small pollution sources, such as dry cleaners. The EPA was committed to the ASPEN model even when compelling community-generated information suggested that it might not accurately characterize local air toxics exposures. As street scientists generate maps that reframe and reorient definitions of "problems," and as these same scientists develop the sophisticated skills of computer-aided mapping, they will continue to blur the line between professional and local knowledge and whose evidence counts as credible in environmental health decision making.

Street Science: Toward Environmental Health Justice

Learning from Community Scientists

Everyday, in neighborhoods across the country, community residents are doing *street science*. They are acting on hypotheses—often developed over years of living with environmental pollution and disease—organizing community insights, employing professional techniques, and fundamentally altering the way environmental-health science is practiced. The residents in Brooklyn have shown that street science is crucial for achieving environmental-health justice—eliminating inequitable exposure and disease burdens, and democratizing research and intervention decision making. Whenever professionals are hesitant to involve local people, especially the poor and people of color, concerned community residents will continue to perform their science in the streets.

The kind of information that street scientists offer varies—from missing hazard information to detailed cultural practices that influence human exposures to pollution—but this knowledge is as much "expertise" as the information that professionals offer. The four episodes detailed in this book reveal that expertise is a crucial political resource in science-intensive policy disputes, since access to knowledge and the ability to question the data that are used to legitimize decisions are essential sources of power and influence. The episodes suggest that political power hinges in part on the ability to manipulate knowledge and to challenge evidence presented in support of particular policies. Ultimately, expertise, whether called professional or local, is a political resource exploited to justify political decisions; it is not an objective truth.

The work of street scientists, it should be clear, is not inherently superior to nor should it always replace professional ways of knowing and acting. Rather, the boundaries placed around problems, the alternatives weighed, and the issues regarded as important tend to determine which "knowledge" is important. The greatest challenge facing *street scientists* is not deciding whether professional or local knowledge is more appropriate, but rather how to recognize, based on the problem being addressed, new modes of collaborative inquiry that can capture the contributions from both local and professional science to improve environmental health for all. The persistence of this challenge, beyond the episodes presented here from one Brooklyn neighborhood, makes clear that these are not unique events. Street scientists are part of a significant movement to reassess the priorities and political relationships that shape environmental-health decision making.

Challenges to Street Science

Studies of local knowledge and community-based practices, particularly in environmental-health politics, often are challenged for romanticizing local culture and practice and overlooking the structural and global dimensions of problem solving. For example, skeptics might accuse this book of being too sympathetic to "identity groups," and in the process reifying social divisions among groups. This critique claims that valorizing identity groups as important sources of knowledge and political claims perpetuates divisions among social groups that are often creations of the State.

A similar critique might label this work "populism" since it challenges elitist notions that ordinary people cannot think or act as rationally as experts. Critics might emphasize that populism also is associated with a reactionary antielitism that has been challenged on a number of fronts, including being called anti-intellectualist (sometimes undercutting rational debate by discarding logic and factual evidence in favor of following the emotional appeals of demagogues), majoritarian (emphasizing that the will of the majority of people has absolute primacy in matters of governance, often sacrificing rights for minorities), moralistic (evangelical-style campaigns sometimes leading to authoritarian and theocratic attempts to impose orthodoxy, especially relating to gender), and nationalistic (patriotic nationalism often promoting ethnocentric, nativist, or xenophobic fears that immigrants and ethnic and religious minorities bring alien ideas and customs that are harmful to "white culture"). Populist political movements also are criticized for "get the government off my back" economic libertarianism, xenophobia and ethnocentric nationalism, scapegoating, and for assuming that "the people" are united in rejecting ordinary politics in favor of spontaneous popular revolution (Canovan 1981; Kazin 1995).

Finally, this research might be challenged for exonerating the State's responsibility to protect those least well-off and shifting the burden of gathering information to local people. This same critique suggests that emphasizing local knowledge ignores the social, political, and economic structures and institutions that help create the environmental burdens currently facing the poor and people of color. These critics might understand local knowledge as parochial and condemned to "the neighborhood," and this, they say, ignores national and global politics.

These challenges raise a number of questions that this concluding chapter attempts to address, including: Do lay people, by entering into the domains of and engaging with professional science, run the risk of being exploited? What institutional decision-making arrangements are necessary to ensure local expertise is considered appropriately? How can local knowledge help reveal how structural inequalities manifest themselves in everyday life? If local knowledge helps reveal the assumptions of professional science, how can we ensure that local knowledge is subject to equally intense scrutiny? Do lay people and social movements reproduce the same type of unequal distribution of knowledge and authoritative claims-making that often plagues professional institutions? How can local groups manage internal tensions that may arise when balancing participating in the construction of scientific knowledge and building and maintaining social and political movements? Some generalizable lessons from the four cases address these critiques and questions.

Street Science and Political Power

For "outsiders," such as planners, to effectively incorporate *street science* into their work, they first must understand residents' experiences, appreciate the nuances in what residents are saying, and be willing to work with residents in formulating policy responses that take account of both professional judgment and local knowledge (Gaventa 1993). This will not happen easily. Professionals remain skeptical of local knowledge and almost always will find it easier to defer to the politically powerful knowledge of private-interest groups or other professional scientists (Bunders and Leydesdorff 1987). Yet, as the cases in this book have shown, *street science* can challenge the "dominant system" by entering the domain of professionals while simultaneously deconstructing professional ideas and methods as inadequate representations of the sum total of reality. Part of the political power of street scientists comes when they enter the terrain of professionals and challenge conventional ways of framing problems, employing methods, and using knowledge in decision making. Since local people generally are at a disadvantage in processes that judge scientific credibility, they often must organize social movements, find ways to "hitch" their ideas to other social-justice issues, and use intermediaries to gain standing in the claims-making process. The Brooklyn activists' street science reveals at least four policy conditions that will help address, but not eliminate, power imbalances between *street scientists* and professionals:

Coalition Formation   Local residents mobilizing into a community coalition in order to gather information and influence professionals.

Issue Linkage   The street science of community residents is linked to a larger social movement outside the community and can scale up to broader policy frames.

Intermediaries   Entrepreneurs or boundary spanners assist local people in the street science process and help them translate what they know for professionals.

Effective Interventions   Street scientists are able to identify short-term interventions that both improve community well-being and build toward broader policy changes.

Coalition Formation
The first policy condition posits that *street science* is most likely to confront power imbalances between community members and professionals

when it is part of a local coalition, not just the isolated stories of one individual or even a few individuals. A community coalition can be a loosely coupled group of residents who ban together to investigate a problem or a more formal community-based organization with ties to the neighborhood. Social movements act as organizers of local environmental-health knowledge, give public voice to private suffering, and gain the attention of elected officials and other policy professionals (Mansbridge 1986). For instance, in the Woburn case made famous by the book and film *A Civil Action*, local people were able to make their concerns known and attract the attention of environmental regulators only after a concerned mother named Anne Anderson organized concerned residents into the coalition *For a Cleaner Environment (FACE)* (Brown and Mikkelsen 1990; Harr 1996). Brown (1993) notes that Anderson asked the State to test the water in Woburn after she collected stories of neighbors whose children had developed cancer but was told the State could not test the water at an individual's initiative. However, when FACE made a similar request, the State listened. Community coalitions are important not only for influencing professionals but also for building the supportive and trusting social networks that proved so crucial for street scientists in Brooklyn.

The formation of local knowledge "advocacy" coalitions is one way that street science might influence professionals (Jenkins-Smith and Sabatier 1997). In this view, State or professional knowledge reflects the politically powerful knowledge coalition. As Kingdon (1984) and Reich (1991) have pointed out, the complexity of modern government not only makes it difficult for the lone amateur to learn what is going on, whom to contact, and where to go to get information, but ordinary citizens also must compete against well-organized interest groups (e.g., business lobbyists and trade associations). Civic coalitions organized into social movements can influence professionals by changing the terms of political discourse (i.e., civil-rights movements), establishing a permanent place on the political agenda for issues (i.e., feminism's raising awareness of gender relations), organizing alternative policy-oriented deliberative forums (i.e., environmental-justice networks), and creating the fear of political instability and therefore drawing forth governmental response (Piven and Cloward 1979).

El Puente's work in Brooklyn is one of the strongest examples of effective community mobilization. The strong local capacity-building and community-organizing effort helped El Puente reach thousands of residents in its door-to-door surveys and focus-group discussions. The information the group gathered was clearly credible science and helped extend the work of conventional science. Yet, as the group engaged in the highly uncertain arena of environmental-health science, the information gathered challenged their original hypothesis that air pollution was the primary cause of asthma. The group had to reflect internally about the causal stories it would use in its community-organizing efforts. El Puente's research contributed to new knowledge about local asthma, but it also raised questions about the representations of the disease they were offering in street protests. Street scientists inevitably will confront this dilemma when engaging with professionals in environmental-health research.

Issue Linkage

Closely related to the importance of community-based coalitions, linking street science to a larger social movement also makes it more likely to influence professionals. Scaling up local issues to broader policy issues often is predicated on the existence of a local coalition. An example of issue linkage and scale-up is how grassroots antitoxics campaigns linked up with civil rights movements to create the environmental-justice movement (Dowie 1995; Schlosberg 1999). More recently, local environmental-justice activists in California joined with immigrant and human-rights groups to influence the Sierra Club when the national environmental group considered opposing immigration.[55] In another example of issue linkage, the coalition Just Transition brought together the Oil, Chemical, and Atomic Workers Union with community-based environmental organizations in order to shape public policy that simultaneously protects workers and the poor communities that surround industrial facilities (Burrows 2001; Rose 2000).[56] In yet another example, a successful campaign against female genital mutilation was a result of organizers' ability to frame the problem as one of human rights and violence to women and "hitched" it to the global human and women's rights movements. In each instance, a local issue is reframed as a piece of a larger social, economic, or political justice campaign.

Street scientists are building international coalitions in order to influence global environment, development, and trade decisions that impact local communities. For example, a coalition of grassroots native-rights groups that make up the Indigenous Environmental Network and other local indigenous-people organizations from around the world have formed the Indigenous Mining Campaign Project in order to share knowledge about sustainable natural-resource and land-management practices and to challenge the mining practices of multinational corporations.[57] Indigenous activists also have organized into a network that has made respecting and protecting their knowledge and information-collection processes a key issue for international organizations such as the World Trade Organization and the World Health Organization.

The World Social Forum has become the place where local knowledges are shared among activists concerned with scaling up what they know into a global social-justice agenda. These local activists have highlighted how international treaty-making over biodiversity, bioprospecting, and intellectual-property rights must take account of local knowledge and respect traditional natural-resource practices (Laird 2002). These examples point to how local knowledge is already scaling-up and playing an important role in reshaping global environmental and public-health decision making.

However, for local coalitions to link up successfully with and hitch onto national and global social movements, community members must explore allegiances with organizations that may not be in their traditional networks. Granovetter (1973) noted that weak ties are more important than strong ties among groups because when organizations are tightly coupled and interact frequently, ideas and information are recirculated through the network. However, the interaction of organizations with "weak ties" (organizations having few overlapping interests and infrequent contact) offers, a greater possibility for new information to be passed between groups (Granovetter 1973).[58] Street scientists should explore the weak ties in their networks to form the broad-based coalitions needed to link local knowledge with global struggles.

The Watchperson Project tied the dietary aspect of the community-exposure-assessment project to larger discussions about cumulative-risk assessment, environmental justice, and the economic and social conditions facing urban immigrants. The group was successful in convincing the EPA to let them survey anglers largely because they argued that in order to capture honest information about angler practices, surveyors first had to understand the conditions of poverty and cultural practices in which fish diets were embedded. The result was that people of color, immigrants, and other non-English speakers performed the interviews and helped analyze the data—a significant challenge to professional research methods.

The lead poisoning episode revealed the importance of both local coalition building and issue linkage. WABBA's intra- and inter-community coalition building around childhood lead poisoning was a key factor in its initial success influencing professionals to address the potential hazards from the bridge sand blasting operation. This community coalition of local residents, local neighborhood organizations, groups from neighborhoods around the Williamsburg Bridge in Manhattan, and organizations concerned with lead poisoning more generally tapped into the strength of a national movement to make their issues heard. The coalition had publicized studies of childhood lead poisoning in the city, built a broad-based coalition, and hitched itself to the national effort to end childhood lead poisoning. As a result of this issue-linkage, WABBA gained significant influence with professionals early on in the controversy. The City agreed to soil remediation, street sweeping, and a blood-lead screening program and invited coalition members to the task force created to address the controversy.

Similarly, El Puente was successful in gathering information about home remedies because it linked its asthma work to challenge assumptions about gendered roles in the Latino community. El Puente hired unemployed women from the neighborhood to perform much of the surveying, data analysis, and focus-group work. During community discussions of home remedies, the El Puente health workers gave a prominent role to folk healers—often elderly women who did not speak English. While these healers are recognized and respected in the Latino community, they are rarely given a public voice. By placing women at the center of their asthma research and intervention, El Puente challenged conventional assumptions about the role of women in the Latino community and also the role of women (including folk healers) in contributing to professional environmental-health knowledge. The larger point here is that if the local knowledge of oppressed people is gathered but reflects racist or sexist positions, it will ultimately fail to resonate with both local people and outside professionals. A key lesson is that the mobilization of street science by community coalitions is more likely to be successful when linked to more general struggles against social inequalities.

Embedded within street science is the opportunity to challenge prevailing hierarchies of power. As Iris Young (1996) has noted, mobilizing local knowledge has the potential to reveal the "particular experiences" of groups in social locations; these experiences are not known by groups "situated differently," but these differently situated groups must understand the experiences of the "other" in order for justice to be served. In this way, local knowledge helps "unmask" how individuals in disadvantaged communities experience inequality, and it can help those not experiencing inequality but are in positions to alleviate suffering better understand the ways this might be accomplished. Local knowledge, and the street science upon which it is based, is unlikely to be influential for those within or outside the community in the long run unless it has an explicit link to other social-justice struggles.

Intermediaries

Street science is more likely to confront professional power when an intermediary or entrepreneur—an institution or agent who can champion and translate local information in professional terms—is present. Intermediaries can be professionals themselves or effective local people affiliated with a respected institution. Professionals often need "translators" because the value of local knowledge to their work and institutional commitments may not be obvious at first glance. Intermediaries do not speak for local people, but merely work to increase the "standing" of what they have described. Effective intermediaries, like street scientists, must hold a "double consciousness," of both the local and professional understanding of problems. That is, intermediaries must have the language, skills, and "cultural capital" to be accepted as legitimate in both local and professional circles.

Intermediaries also can be thought of as "boundary spanners"—individuals and organizations with sufficient power and resources to move ideas, information, and organizational legitimacy across institutional boundaries (Aldrich and Herker 1977; Tushman and Scanlan 1981; DiMaggio and Powell 1991). According to organizational theory, boundary spanning is intended to address uncertainty and indeterminacy in decision making by increasing coordination and interdependence among stakeholders and organizations (Aldrich and Herker 1977).

The subsistence fishing and asthma episodes highlight that community groups may be most effective using intermediaries when street scientists engage in community-based research partnerships with professionals. The Watchperson Project partnered with the EPA to develop their angler survey and interview protocol, and the agency helped gather toxicological data and estimate cancer risks from ingestion rates derived from the community research. El Puente partnered with Community Information and Epidemiological Technologies to learn how to design and administer a survey, interpret data, and train community-health workers. In both instances, community residents helped frame research questions, define problems, decide what information would count, and choose the credible sources of useful data. In these processes, community members act alongside scientists as equal partners in problem definition, information collection, and data analysis—all geared toward locally relevant action for social change (Israel et al. 1998; Minkler 2000).

However, communities need to engage intermediaries with caution. Recall that the major failure in the lead-poisoning case was that WABBA could not articulate its knowledge, stories, and experience into coherent knowledge, and the intermediaries they hired failed to help them do this. While intermediaries can be effective translating local knowledge for outsiders when community groups have developed a clear statement of what they want and what they have found, they can be detrimental when they offer conflicting advice or when community groups do not have an organized process for managing the tensions that arise.

The street-science process creates a challenging dilemma for local groups. In community-based environmental-health controversies, politically vulnerable groups of lay people are likely to be dependent on and potentially antagonistic to the same group of professionals. The complexity of this dynamic should not be underestimated. Community groups often recognize their dependence on a group of professionals (e.g., scientists) for helping them solve the problems they face but may also blame this same group of experts for contributing to their predicament in the first place. The work of Brooklyn activists highlights that intermediaries can enable, as in the case of the Watchperson Project, or stymie, as in the lead-poisoning case, the efforts of street scientists in confronting professional power.

Effective Interventions

A fourth condition for *street science* to confront power is efficient and effective interventions that improve short-term health and environmental conditions, but also are linked to broader social policies. This proposition is based on Kingdon's notion of a "policy stream" in which a policy response is "waiting" for the articulation of a social problem (Kingdon 1984). For example, the passage of the Montreal Protocol limiting the production and use of ozone-depleting chemicals has been attributed to the ready availability of substitute chemicals (Benedick 1998). Of course, many interventions can have displacement effects, for example shipping toxic waste for cheap disposal in a developing country, smokestacks reducing local pollution but polluting farther away, and the drying and burning of sewage turning a water pollution problem into air pollution. The aim is to avoid interventions that displace the locus of power and to resist shifting the burden of proof or generation of interventions to those already bearing the brunt of society's ills.

Since communities confronting environmental-health problems can't wait for definitive proof of environmental-health threats before taking action, an effective intervention for local people means taking action in the face of incomplete information and uncertainty. Precautionary interventions can address the short-term feelings of powerlessness many low-income populations and communities of color feel regarding improving community health. Precautionary action also is an important way to learn about how to intervene more effectively, particularly when social learning is built into the evaluation of interventions. Under conditions of social learning, organizations can alter actions as new information emerges.

El Puente's work provides perhaps the best examples of effective short-term interventions linked to broader policy action. When the organization learned that many low-income Latinos did not have health insurance, residents were enrolled in a free New York State health-insurance program. When later interviews and surveys revealed that residents often decided whether to visit a physician for asthma care based not on the availability of health care but whether they *trusted* their physicians, El Puente changed its focus. The group developed a "cultural competency" program for physicians and other professionals at a local hospital and, at the same time, organized focus groups and a new survey to capture more information about physician distrust. The subsequent survey and focus groups revealed the widespread use of home remedies, which often replaced prescribed medications. Based on this finding, the group added another intervention strategy aimed at exploring ways to integrate herbal and home remedies with physician-prescribed medications in asthma management plans. Eventually this effort gained resonance with professionals, as evidenced by the fact that El Puente's cultural competency training program received funding from the National Institute of Environmental Health Sciences.

Taking short-term precautionary actions that build toward broad policy changes also helps highlight, for both community residents and professionals, that *street science* is no panacea for solving environmental-health problems. Just as community members reject professional science as not the sum total of reality, so too should street science be scrutinized and viewed as partial; no one "truth" or worldview is capable of addressing complex environmental health problems. When *street science* is included in decision-making debates, it too can be deconstructed, scrutinized, and understood for its strengths and weaknesses. The street science of Brooklyn activists revealed that local knowledge was crucial for addressing some problems, such as neighborhood-level hazardous exposures, but these same problems also require action at regional, national, and international levels. Taking contingent action informed by local knowledge emphasizes, perhaps contrary to intuition, that professional science and the State must remain major players in environmental-health problem solving. Although *street science* has its limits, it suggests that the State's appropriate role is enabling, facilitating, supporting, and responding to local initiatives rather than always imposing initiatives of its own.

Street Science and Environmental-Health Practice

This book has argued that when professionals fail to acknowledge the value street science brings to environmental-health decision making, their work misses important information, is less effective, and is less democratic. Yet, local knowledge is not something that professionals likely will be able to acquire on their own, even those who may be committed to fusing street science with their professional work. *Street science* is not merely a set of methods and techniques that anyone can learn with enough attention and practice. Rather, it is as much a process as it is particular information. Even if professionals understood the local knowledge in a particular place or community and how to gather it, they could not necessarily export this insight to another "place" or community without going through the processes associated with *street science*. The processes communities use to mobilize knowledge, including organizing coalitions, gathering and sharing information, assessing options for action, and building partnerships with professionals, all suggest that *street science* is something that never can be ignored by professionals concerned with both using the best available science and achieving democratic decision making.

Street science also can speak to professional concerns, particularly those of urban planners and spatial epidemiologists, about how the qualities of places and the "built environment" are linked to the health of populations. For professionals the dominant models for intervention remain policy sectors (e.g., transportation, housing, environment, public health, etc.), largely constructed from economic and social-policy objectives. Distinct functions have been privileged in regulation over the interconnection of multiple activities in regions, communities, and neighborhoods.

The insights from street scientists have revealed the importance of local context and that the dominant regulatory modes are providing inadequate protection for disadvantaged populations. For example, the current regulatory framework presumes that environmental laws are geographically neutral; they should apply equally everywhere, within the relevant jurisdiction, and therefore advances in protecting the environment should benefit everyone equally. Yet, the inattention to geographic place may limit the current environmental-management system from addressing the community-based hazards raised here. Current environmental regulations focus primarily on three methods of hazard management. The first approach is to control the activity causing the pollution (e.g., energy production, agriculture, transportation), and, the EPA regulates by industrial sector. A second approach is to target an agent or specific pollutant (e.g., lead, asbestos, radon), a scenario usually only used to control perceived immediate threats to human health. The third and most widely used approach targets the medium or, less frequently, the route of exposure (e.g., drinking water, ambient air, pesticides on food). Environmental problems in the current regulatory system rarely are defined or addressed as place-based issues.

The Brooklyn street scientists have highlighted the importance of place-based knowledge for understanding and effectively addressing environmental-health problems. The knowledge of geographic place was crucial for understanding particular local environmental exposures, including where anglers caught fish for subsistence diets, the types of employment available for local Latinas, and the location of small-source air polluters, such as the dry cleaners in residential buildings the Watchperson Project identified. When professionals begin to consider street science, they will understand better the characteristics of a place and learn from locals how to tailor interventions that most effectively address the needs of a place and the diverse populations in urban neighborhoods.

Street Science Encouraging the "Jazz of Practice"

This book began with a suggestion that professionals ought to stop seeing themselves as static purveyors of a technical rationality (or any specific rationality for that matter) and instead engage critically with the tensions and contradictions that are inherent to their own decision making and in the thinking of the publics they are supposed to serve. In short, professionals ought to become, borrowing from Donald Schon (1983), "reflexive practitioners." The case studies have shown that professionals must make new commitments in their work in order to understand the insights of populations suffering from disproportionate environmental exposure and disease burdens and to enable, not stymie, the work of street scientists. This type of practice will likely be unfamiliar terrain for most professionals. Therefore, a metaphor of something familiar—jazz— can best describe this new ideal professional practice.

Jazz music is about improvisation, creativity, and building a group sound. The jazz musician builds on and responds to the actions and tones of other musicians in the group. While the musician reacts in the moment, she does not enter the "jam session" unprepared or without a repertoire of responses. Jazz musicians have a keen sense of history— the origins of the music, those who came before them, and the riffs and arrangements that define the genre. In the *jazz of practice*, professionals will bring their conventional "tool kit" but be rewarded for improvising and being creative. They also will be encouraged to forge new partnerships and to be open to new interpretations of seemingly routine situations.

While jazz is largely about improvisation, accepted rules of procedure exist—when to solo, how to yield to another musician, when to break with tone and how to "bring back the rhythm." It is untrue that anything goes. In the *jazz of practice*, professionals still will bring their disciplinary methods, but they also must learn and respect the rules and norms—the everyday rhythms—of the cultures and communities with whom they work.

Finally, jazz music emerged out of the struggle by African-Americans for recognition and equality. To be a jazz musician is to embody and continue the struggle for justice, racial equality, and an end to all discrimination. In the *jazz of practice*, professionals are expected to situate themselves in this struggle and make this a centerpiece of their work. By being playful, improvisational, and open to new "players," the *jazz of practice* encourages professionals to reinvent and remake existing models of environmental-health decision making.

Toward Environmental Health Justice

Street science is no panacea. Yet, when street science identifies hazards, highlights previously ignored questions, provides hard-to-gather data, involves difficult-to-reach populations, and expands the possibilities for intervention alternatives, science and democracy are improved. When *street science* is meaningfully considered by professionals, they are more likely to understand the claims made by the publics they are supposed to serve—and these same publics are more likely to, in turn, trust the professionals. Improved trust is likely to ease the work of professionals and allay community fears that interventions are not addressing their priorities.

Fundamentally, *street science* is about the pursuit of environmental-health justice. Mobilizing local knowledge helps disadvantaged communities organize and educate themselves, as well as increases control over the decisions that impact their lives. Communities also benefit from the mobilization of street science by shifting the environmental discourse from protest and refusal to engagement with problem solving. Community groups can use street science to complement other actions they may be involved in, such as lawsuits. Finally, street science pursues environmental-health justice by explicitly valuing the different rituals of learning that communities use to understand, analyze, and act upon the problems they face. Figure 7.1 summarizes some of the ways *street science* contributes to the professional and community pursuit of environmental health justice.

The main goal of this book was to contribute to a better descriptive, analytic, and prescriptive understanding of local environmental-health knowledge. The work of Brooklyn's street scientists has shown that solving environmental-health problems in today's deindustrialized urban neighborhoods requires rich contextual knowledge often unattainable by outsiders. While capable of becoming competent scientists in their own right, the residents in these areas face the additional burdens of obscene levels of poverty and racial segregation that persist in many cities across the United States. Yet, like the jazz funeral that mourns death in its first line and celebrates life in its second, *street science* encourages both the repulsion of dominant modes of professional rationality while optimistically attempting to restructure professional–local interactions toward more democratic environmental-health decision making. The case for street science is strong; improved scientific information, a method for community organizing, and a way to ensure interventions are contextually relevant. As the health and well-being of disenfranchised urban residents and their neighborhoods hangs in the balance, street scientists are proving that environmental-health decisions can be more democratic, more just, and more protective for everyone.

How *Street Science* Pursues Environmental Health Justice

Helping professionals:
• **Identifies hazards**   reveal some problems that professionals may have missed and raise new questions about hazards that matter most to those most impacted by hazard exposures.
• **Provides good data**   some information is inaccessible to outsiders; professional data is always partial and sketchy.
• **Improves access to difficult-to-reach informants/clients**   local knowledge can make reluctant community members, such as immigrants and non-English speakers, participate and can overcome disincentives to participation, such as poverty.
• **Expands scope of implementation alternatives**   "expands the pie" of considerations for interventions.
• **Improves implementation success**   by recognizing various actors, perspectives, practices and traditions that influence the effectiveness of local policy.
• **Increases understanding of community claims**   in order to work well with communities, professionals need to understand what residents think, what they do, and what they want, and *street science* is one way to organize this information.
• **Increases trust and credibility**   with skeptical publics.
• **Recognizes the fallibility of local knowledge**   incorporating local knowledge into public debate, opens it up to scrutiny, criticism and testing.

Helping communities:
• **Organizing**   build community coalitions through production and sharing of information, practices, and images.
• **Empowerment**   educate, raise awareness, and develop self-help strategies through mobilization of knowledge and action strategies.
• **Recognition**   residents have important information, can be trusted, are not ignorant, and are not dependent on professionals for problem solving.
• **Improves intra-community decision-making**   provides new information for local groups to help themselves, define priority issues and learn what is important to constituents.
• **Enhance community control**   local knowledge mobilization, organizing and local decision-making are all attempts by disadvantaged groups to enhance control over their own lives.
• **Shifts environmental discourse**   from protest and refusal to positive demands and engagement in problem solving.
• **Supplements other actions**   *street science* can contribute to other problem-solving strategies such as lawsuits.
• **Rituals of learning**   *street science* mobilization legitimizes alternative ways of learning about problems, such as through story-telling, visual images, theatrical performance, and community tours.

Figure 7.1.
How *street science* pursues environmental-health justice.

Notes

Many of the quotations in this book are from the author's personal communications, conversations, and meeting notes. Many of the individuals wished to remain anonymous.

1. The World Health Organization defines "health" as "a state of complete physical, mental, and social well-being and not merely the absence of disease or infirmity." www.who.int/aboutwho/en/definition.html

2. I borrow the idea of "scaling up" from the work of Derthick (1999).

3. Jasanoff (1999) and others note that in Europe, the precautionary principle is another way to frame environmental problems. Tesh (2000) also notes that the discourse of risk in environmental-health policy shifted the focus of regulation from eliminating harms to managing risks.

4. A series of additional ideological and methodological challenges to risk assessment are described in detail in chapter 3.

5. In general, the book aims to avoid suggesting that all professionals act a certain way in all situations, just as it avoids essentializing what lay people know and do in all situations. The book highlights dominant tendencies and seeks to uncover why these trajectories persist rather than assume that all members of particular groups act similarly.

6. It is useful to be clear about what I mean by knowledge. I accept the definition of knowledge as "the state or fact of knowing; familiarity, awareness, or understanding gained through experience or study; the sum or range of what has been perceived, discovered, or learned; learning; erudition; specific information about something" (American Heritage Dictionary, Second college edition).

7. Levi-Straus, comments on definitions of local knowledge this way: "The thought we call primitive is founded on this demand for order. This is equally true of all thought but it is through the properties common to all thought that we can most easily begin to understand all forms of thought which seem very strange to us" (1962, 10).

8. *Indigenous Knowledge and Development Monitor* 1(2). June 1993. www .nuffic.nl/ciran/ikdm/1-2/contents.html

9. This story comes from Irwin 1995.

10. This story comes primarily from Epstein 1996.

11. This story comes from interviews with Corbin-Mark (2001) and Northridge (2001), as well as the following published material: Northridge, Vallone, et al. 2000; Kinney 2000; Northridge, Kinney, et al. 2000.

12. The ideas of habitus and cultural capital come from Bourdieu 1977. For Bourdieu, "habitus" refers to the modes of conduct, taste, and feeling which predominate among members of particular groups. It can refer to shared traits of which the people who share them may be largely unconscious. It is very similar to the English expression "second nature," an acquired tendency that has become instinctive. "Cultural capital" might be understood, like social, political, and other forms of capital, as ways of being, acting, speaking, etc., that are considered legitimate in the eyes of the dominant culture.

13. Michael Dyson writes on the need to move beyond essentialism in expanding African-American cultural criticism:

Of course, I don't mean that there are not distinct black cultural characteristics that persist over space and time, but these features of black life are the products of the historical and social construction of racial identity. . . . These distinct features of black life nuance and shape black cultural expression, from the preaching of Martin Luther King to the singing of Gladys Knight. They do not, however, form the basis of a black racial or cultural essence. Nor do they indicate that *the* meaning of blackness will be expressed in a quality or characteristic without which a person, act, or practice no longer qualifies as black. Rigid racial essentialism must be opposed. (1993, xxi)

14. Krimsky notes that folk wisdom has contributed to technical knowledge through:

pragmatic knowledge obtained through the intergenerational transmission of trail-error experiences, intuitive understanding of complex interactive systems, the generation of scientific hypotheses, and causal links such as identification of the environmental sources of human disease or ecological degradation and an understanding of meaning and value of urban life. (1984, 253)

15. Forester also highlights the idea of "making sense together" by exploring how designers design as much "in their head" as in communication with others (1989, 119–133).

16. "Creating value" is a term borrowed from the negotiation literature and suggests that problem solving is not a "zero sum" game (i.e., what I win, you lose because there is a fixed amount of gains to be had between the two of us). Instead, "creating value" implies that the "pie of gains can be enlarged" (Raiffa 1982).

17. This concept has also been termed "post-normal" science (Funtowicz and Ravetz 1999). The term "post-normal" provides a contrast to two sorts of "normality." One is the picture of research science as "normally" consisting of puzzle solving within the framework of an unquestioned and unquestionable "paradigm," in the theory of Kuhn (1962). Another is the assumption that the policy

environment is "normal" in that routine puzzle solving by experts provides an adequate knowledge base for policy decisions. The idea of post-normal science is to bring "facts" and "values" into a unified conception of problem-solving where a plurality of legitimate perspectives are recognized as capable of contributing to addressing any given problem (Ravetz 1999).

18. For an understanding of "field," I draw from Bourdieu and Wacquant (1992), who describe fields as specific, relatively autonomous, domains of social action, social production and reproduction, which both reflect and constrain the interests, positions, strategies, and investments of the actors within them. While this idea is helpful to understand how lay people attempt to locate themselves within science, it may be too narrow because Bourdieu portrays scientific practice as something carried out in laboratories, universities and peer-reviewed journals, not in social movements.

19. Another major outcome of the DOJ hearing was an investigation by the National Environmental Justice Advisory Council, a Federal Advisory Committee to the EPA, on the civil rights implications of the location and siting practices for waste transfer stations (NEJAC 2000). I explore this meeting in more detail in chapter 6.

20. EPA official interviewed on condition of anonymity.

21. This brief discussion comes from the National Forum on Contaminants in Fish, May 6–9 2001. www.epa.gov/ost/fish/forum/fishforum.pdf

22. The following accounts come from the author's interviews with anglers, most of whom were interviewed by the Watchperson Project during the survey project. Since the interviews conducted during the Watchperson Project survey were not recorded, I chose to interview anglers to recapture these stories for this analysis.

23. These anglers requested that I not use their last names. Interviewed October 14, 2000.

24. I will return to the details of the incinerator story in chapter 6.

25. Atopy is defined as a tendency to immediate hypersensitivity (allergic) reactions involving certain familial conditions such as hay fever, asthma and atopic dermatitis (Pearce, Douwes, and Beasley 2000).

26. Quoted in Stolberg (1999).

27. In an effort not to bias the questionnaire towards asthma, the word asthma does not appear in the survey until question #18, and it is only used if the respondent mentions the term first.

28. Other Hasidim at the meeting who spoke to me on the condition of anonymity, said that a big issue was that all marriages are arranged by family and friends, so if someone knows you have a health problem, even at an early age, you can be stigmatized. They noted that there is a high degree of confidentiality in the community. Christina Lawson, the former director of UJO's Asthma Education Campaign, confirmed this barrier and noted that most people do not speak English well enough to understand or read about health and good translations

into Yiddish do not exist. Lawson also noted that the separation of the sexes required by the Rabbinic Council meant that all survey and education materials had to be reviewed and approved, and, making a survey even more challenging, it was forbidden for men to be alone with a woman unless she was his spouse. All of these dynamics, according to Lawson, contributed to UJO's adamant rejection of the community health survey (Lawson 2001).

29. To put this finding in perspective, the active asthma rate for children in the South Bronx, which has been characterized as having one of the nation's worst childhood asthma problems, is 8.6% (Claudio 1996; Kozol 1995).

30. While the direct health impacts of such a program are hard to measure, a 2000 El Puente survey found that those with management plans were half as likely to have visited a hospital for asthma (Penchaszadeh 2001). While asthma hospitalizations are down city-wide, they have also decreased in Brooklyn Community Board #1 from 1,166 in 1997 to 484 in 1999 (NYC DOH 2000).

31. Important exceptions include critical analyses of planning practice and the role of the professional such as Schon (1983), Forester (1999), and Lee (1993).

32. The lab was International Testing Labs, Inc., of Newark, NJ.

33. Brown and Mikkelson (1990) list the common stages of community mobilization of local environmental health knowledge:

1) People in a contaminated community notice separately both health effects and pollutants.
2) These residents hypothesize something out of the ordinary, typically a connection between the health effects and the pollutants.
3) Community residents share information, creating a common perspective.
4) Community residents, now a more cohesive group, read, ask around, and talk to government officials and scientific experts about the health effects and the putative contaminants.
5) Residents organize groups to pursue their investigation.
6) Government agencies conduct official studies in response to community groups' pressure. These studies usually find no association between the contaminants and health effects.
7) Community groups bring in their own experts to conduct a health study and to investigate pollutant sources and pathways.
8) Community groups engage in litigation and confrontation.
9) Community groups press for corroboration of their findings by official experts and agencies.

They note that each stage is not necessarily completed before the next begins, but the stages usually follow this order.

34. The US EPA has set 10 micrograms per deciliter (mg/dl) as the maximum safe concentration of blood-lead in children under six years of age. Any concentration above 10 is considered lead poisoning. See: "Eliminating Childhood Lead Poisoning: A Federal Strategy Targeting Lead Paint Hazards," President's Task Force on Environmental Health Risks and Safety Risks to Children, February 2000. www.epa.gov/children/whatwe/leadhaz.pdf

35. At the time, the EPA had not set cleanup guidelines for lead contaminated soil.

36. NYC Health Code, § 11.03(a) (1997). Lead poisoning was added to the list of legally reportable diseases on June 16, 1986, and the definition of lead poisoning under this code provision was amended to include all children with blood lead levels of 10 µg/dl or higher on October 6, 1992. The City Health Code is more strict than the State Health Code, 10 N.Y.C.R.R. § 22.7, which is permissible pursuant to Public Health Law § 228.

37. The following details come directly from New York State Supreme Court case documents: *WABBA v Guliani*, Index No. 94/106235. Affidavits and Exhibits in support of petition.

38. Supreme Court of the State of New York, County of New York. Index No. 94/106235. Record of Decision, October 6, 1995.

39. The only two alternatives studied in the EIS were, (1) lead paint removal activity with proposed containment and (2) no paint removal activity but paint weathers and releases into the environment (NYC DOT 1998, 20–22).

40. The Draft EIS stated:

While a handful of data outlier points may have a substantial visual impact, they contribute little to any qualitative measure of an association between bridge proximity and blood lead levels. The EIS uses accepted statistical techniques (regression analysis) to objectively check for the presence of such a trend and none was found. In fact, as stated in the EIS, blood lead levels near the bridge are slightly lower than blood lead levels measured at locations further away on both sides of the bridge. (NYC DOT 1998, 20–49)

41. One parallel political battle was between the Brooklyn Borough President's office and Assemblyman Joseph R. Lentol, Democrat of Brooklyn, both of whom wanted to get credit from their constituencies for helping to stop the bridge sandblasting. A second was a leadership struggle over the Watchperson Project between Deborah Masters and Inez Pasher. A third battle was over the City's funding of a new community advisory committee to oversee the reconstruction of the Newtown Creek Sewage Treatment Plant located in the Greenpoint neighborhood.

42. I was an observer at two of these meetings. The following comments come from my observations and field notes. They also come from written documentation issued at and after the meetings and interviews with key participants.

43. Since the speaker has requested to remain anonymous, I have used a pseudonym.

44. See: www.toxicavenger.com.

45. The main players in the multi-ethnic, multi-racial anti-incinerator coalition were El Puente, UJO, and the Polish and Slavic Center (PSC).

46. The march was called "CAFE con LECHE" because the Brooklyn CAFE coalition marched over the bridge to Manhattan to meet another community coalition opposing the incinerator called, Lower Eastside Coalition for Health and the Environment (LECHE).

47. Under a 1991 court order, DEC and DOS share responsibility for review of solid waste transfer stations under the State Environmental Quality Review Act. DEC leads in review of natural resource issues and DOS in issues of social and economic impact.

48. USA Waste Corporation was later acquired by Waste Management Inc. and the transfer station proposal was also pursued by Waste Management.

49. See: Howard S. Golden, et al. v. Michael Carpinello, et ano, Supreme Court of New York, Index Number 42723/98. Some of the community groups included Neighbors Against Garbage (NAG), Organization of Waterfront Neighborhoods (OWN), Red Hook Civic Association, El Puente, New York City Environmental Justice Alliance, The Watchperson Project, Organizations United for Trash Reduction and Garbage Equity (OUTRAGE) and Boroughs Allied for Recycling and Garbage Equity (BARGE). The case was submitted by the New York Lawyers for the Public Interest and Brooklyn Legal Services.

50. I attended the hearing as a member of the NYC DEP but was not involved in the review of the facility. The following accounts of the meeting are from my notes and observations unless cited otherwise.

51. State of New York, Executive Chamber, Press Office, June 23, 1998. "Governor Pataki, Mayor Giuliani Announce Environmental Review for Brooklyn Transfer Station." Governor Pataki notes in the announcement: "Given the location of both these actions under consideration by the State and the City, and after hearing the community's concerns about this project, we are requiring the preparation of an environmental impact statement."

52. In 2000, Congresswoman Nydia Velazquez filed a Title VI Civil Rights complaint with the EPA, asserting that G/W residents have been targeted for transfer stations. She also introduced the 2001 Community Environmental Equity Act (HR 4939), which prohibited disproportionate exposure to hazardous substances based on race, color, national origin, or economic status. See, www .house.gov/velazquez/PressReleases/2001/pr010420.htm.

53. EPA scientist interviewed on April 24, 2000, on the condition of anonymity.

54. Perc is a dry-cleaning solvent and at high exposures has been shown to have adverse effects on the central nervous system, liver and kidneys. The US EPA Cancer Benchmark Level for Perc is 1.7ppb. A report by the NYC Public Advocate, *Clothed in Controversy II: The Urgent Need to Protect New Yorkers from Toxic Dry Cleaning Fumes*, March 18, 1997, noted that two flights above a dry cleaner in Tribeca, perc levels were measured at 5–16 times the State DOH guideline. See: publicadvocate.nyc.gov/padcdetail.cfm?id1=7&2=46.

55. See: "Anti-immigration policy loses in landslide," www.enn.com/enn-news-archive/1998/04/042798/immivote_21739.asp.

56. See: www.justtransition.org/.

57. The international coalition of indigenous organizations includes: Tebtebba Foundation, African Indigenous Women's Organization, Indigenous Information Network, Asian Indigenous Women's Network, International Indian Treaty

Council, Indigenous Women's Network, Third World Network, Inuit Circumpolar Conference; Asian Indigenous Peoples Pact; Kalipunan ng Mamamayang Katutubo ng Pilipinas (KAMP Philippines), International Alliance of Indigenous and Tribal Peoples of the Tropical Forests; Pastoralists Indigenous Non-Government Organization (Tanzania), Nepalese Indigenous Peoples Development and Information Service Center, Defensa y Conservacion Ecologica de Intag Ecuador DECOIN (Ecuador), and Coordinadora Nacional de Comunidades del Peru Afectadas por la Mineria CONACAMI (Peru).

58. The "strength of weak ties" idea has had a particular resonance in social-network theory. The classic example claims that when job-seekers find work through personal contacts, the referrals come much more often through distant contacts than through more immediate relations. In an example from this case, many environmental activists know one another well, and public health professionals also know one anther well. But few professional public health practitioners know many environmental activists.

References

Abbott, A. 1988. *The system of professions*. Chicago: Chicago University Press.

Abbott, A. 1992. What do cases do? Some notes on activity in sociological analysis. In C. Ragin and H. Becker, *What is a case? Exploring the foundations of social inquiry*. Cambridge: Cambridge University Press.

Aberley, D. 1993. *Boundaries of home: Mapping for local empowerment*. Gabriola Island: New Society Publishers.

Abramson, M., and the Young Lords Party. 1971. *Palante: Young Lords Party*. New York: McGraw-Hill.

Agarwal, A. 1995. Dismantling the divide between indigenous and scientific knowledge. *Development and Change* 26 (3): 413–439.

Agency for Toxic Substances and Disease Registry (ATSDR). 1988. The nature and extent of lead poisoning in children in the United States: A report to Congress. Atlanta: Centers for Disease Control.

Aldrich, H., and Herker, D. 1977. Boundary spanning roles and organizational structure. *Academy of Management Review* 2: 212–229.

American Lung Association (ALA). 1993. Breath in danger, II: Estimation of populations at risk of adverse health consequences in areas not in attainment with national ambient air quality standards of the Clean Air Act. Washington, DC: American Lung Association.

American Thoracic Society (ATS). 1996. Committee of the Environmental and Occupational Health Assembly. Health effects of outdoor air pollution: Part 2. *American Journal of Respiratory and Critical Care Medicine* 153: 477–498.

American Thoracic Society. 2000. What constitutes an adverse health effect of air pollution? *American Journal of Respiratory and Critical Care Medicine* 161: 665–673.

Ames, S. 1998. *Guide to community visioning*. Chicago: American Planning Association Press.

Amy, D. J. 1987. *The politics of environmental mediation*. New York: Columbia University Press.

Anderson, B. 1991. *Imagined communities: Reflections on the origin and spread of nationalism*. Rev. ed. London and New York: Verso.

Anderson, E. 1999. *Code of the street: Decency, violence, and the moral life of the inner city*. New York: Norton & Co.

Argyris, C., and D. A. Schön. 1974. *Theory in practice: Increasing professional effectiveness*. San Francisco: Jossey-Bass.

Argyris, C., and D. A. Schön. 1996. *Organizational learning II: Theory, method, and practice*. Reading, MA: Addison-Wesley.

Arnstein, S. R. 1969. A ladder of citizen participation. *Journal of the American Institute of Planners* 35: 216–224.

Austin, R., and A. Schill. 1994. Black, brown, red, and poisoned. In *Unequal protection: Environmental justice and communities of color*, ed. R. Bullard, 53–74. San Francisco: Sierra Club Books.

Bamberger, L. 1966. Health care and poverty: What are the dimensions of the problem from the community's point of view? *Bulletin of the New York Academy of Medicine* 42: 1140.

Barnett, A. W. 1984. *Community murals: The people's art*. New York: Cornwall Books.

Barnes, B., and D. Bloor. 1982. Relativism, rationalism and the sociology of knowledge. In *Rationality and Relativism*, ed. M. Hollis and S. Lukes, 1–20. Oxford: Basil Blackwell.

Baum, H. S. 1997. *The organization of hope: Communities planning themselves*. Albany: State University of New York.

Beck, U. 1992. *Risk society: Towards a new modernity*. Thousand Oaks, CA: Sage.

Benedick, R. E. 1998. *Ozone diplomacy: New directions in safeguarding the planet*. Cambridge, MA: Harvard University Press.

Benveniste, G. 1972. *The politics of expertise*. Berkeley, CA: Glendessary Press.

Berger, J. 1992. Fear builds a bridge across gulf of cultures. *New York Times*, August 31, B3.

Berkman, L., and I. Kawachi, eds. 2000. *Social epidemiology*. London: Oxford University Press.

Bernstein, R. 1998. Community in the pragmatic tradition. In *The revival of pragmatism*, ed. M. Dickstein. Durham, NC: Duke University Press.

Bourdieu, P. 1977. *Outline of a theory of practice*. Cambridge: Cambridge University Press.

Bourdieu, P. 2000. *Pascalian meditations*. Stanford, CA: Stanford University Press.

Bourdieu, P., and L. Wacquant. 1992. *An invitation to reflexive sociology*. Chicago: University of Chicago Press.

Bragg, R. 1997. Pollution drives away neighborhood and trust. *New York Times*. March 16, A16.

Breyer S. 1993. *Breaking the vicious circle: Toward effective risk regulation.* Cambridge, MA: Harvard University Press.

Brint, S. 1994. *In an age of experts.* Princeton, NJ: Princeton, University Press.

Brown, P. 1987. Popular epidemiology: Community response to toxic waste induced disease in Woburn, Massachusetts, and other sites. *Science, Technology, and Human Values,* 12 (3–4): 76–85.

Brown, P. 1992. Popular epidemiology and toxic waste contamination: Lay and professional ways of knowing. *Journal of Health and Social Behavior* 33: 267–281.

Brown, P. 1993. When the public knows better: Popular epidemiology challenges the system. *Environment* 35 (8): 16–21.

Brown, P. 1997. Popular epidemiology revisited. *Current Sociology* 45 (3): 137–156.

Brown, P., and E. J. Mikkelsen. 1990. *No safe place: Toxic waste, leukemia, and community action.* Berkeley: University of California Press.

Brown, L. D., and R. Tandon. 1983. Ideology and political economy in inquiry: Action research and participatory research. *Journal of Applied Behavioral Science* 19: 277–294.

Brush, S. 1980. Potato taxonomies in Andean agriculture. In *Indigenous knowledge systems and development,* ed. D. Brokensha, D. Warren, and O. Werner, 37–47. Lanham, MD: University Press of America.

Bryant B. 1995. Pollution prevention and participatory research as methodology for environmental justice. *Virginia Environmental Law Journal* 14: 589–612.

Bryant, B., and P. Mohai, eds. 1992. *Race and the incidence of environmental hazards.* Boulder, CO: Westview Press.

Buege, D. 1996. The ecologically noble savage revisited. *Environmental Ethics* 18 (1): 71–88.

Bullard, R. D. 1990. *Dumping in Dixie: Race, class and environmental quality.* Boulder, CO: Westview.

Bullard, R. 1994. *Unequal protection: Environmental justice and communities of color.* San Francisco: Sierra Club Books.

Bullard, R., and G. S. Johnson. 2000. Environmental justice: Grassroots activism and its impact of public policy decision making. *Journal of Social Issues* 56 (3): 555–578.

Bunders, J., and L. Leydesdorff. 1987. The causes and consequences of collaborations between scientists and non-scientific groups. In *The social direction of the public sciences: Causes and consequences of co-operation between scientists and non-scientific groups,* ed. S. Blume, J. Bunders, L. Leydesdorff, and R. Whitley, 331–347. Dordrecht, Holland: Reidel.

Burger, J., K. Staine, and M. Gochfeld. 1993. Fishing in contaminated waters: Knowledge and risk perception of hazards by fishermen in New York City. *Journal of Toxicology and Environmental Health* 39 (1): 95–105.

Burnham, A. C. 1920. *The community health problem.* New York: Macmillan Co.

Burrows, M. 2001. Just transition: Moving to a green economy. *Alternatives Journal* 27: 29–32.

Calderone J., K. Flynn, T. Robbins, and R. Sugarman. 1998. Asthma: The silent epidemic. *New York Daily News*, special series. February 22–26.

Calhoun, C. 1994. *Social theory and the politics of identity*. Cambridge, MA: Blackwell.

Callon, M. 1986. Some elements of a sociology of translation: Domestication of the scallops and fishermen of St. Brieuc Bay. In *Power, action, and belief: A new sociology of knowledge?* ed. J. Law, 196–233. London: Routledge.

Campbell, S. 1996. Green cities, growing cities, just cities? *Journal of the American Planning Association* 62 (3): 296–313.

Canovan, M. 1981. *Populism*. New York: Harcourt Brace Jovanovich.

Carpenter A. 1999. Modern hygiene's dirty tricks. *Science News* 156:108–110.

Carr, W., L. Zeitel, and K. Weiss. 1992. Variations in asthma hospitalizations and deaths in New York City. *American Journal of Public Health* 82: 59–65.

Carroll, M. 1983. Studies criticize New York's plan to burn refuse: Release of dioxins in air called a health threat (City Comptroller Harrison J. Goldin vs. Mayor Koch on Brooklyn Navy Yard incinerator) *New York Times*, (Jan. 24, 12[N], B2[L]).

Centers for Disease Control and Prevention (CDC). 1997. Public Health Practice Program Office. Principles of community engagement. Atlanta, Georgia.

Centers for Disease Control and Prevention (CDC). 1991. Preventing lead poisoning in young children: A statement by the Centers for Disease Control. Atlanta: U.S. Department of Health and Human Services. DHHS Report No. 99-2230.

Centro Internacional de Epidemiología Tropical (CIET). 2000. Available at http://www.ciet.org/www/image/country/_new-frames.html.

Chambers R. 1992. Rural appraisal: Rapid, relaxed, and participaton. Discussion Paper 311. Brighton, England: Institute of Development Studies.

Chambers, R. 1997. *Whose reality counts? Putting the first last*. London: ITDG Publishing.

Chriss, J. J. 1995. Habermas, Goffman, and communicative action: Implications for professional practice. *American Sociological Review* 60: 545–565.

Clark, R., N. B. Anderson, V. R. Clark, and D. R. Williams. 1999. Racism as a stressor for African Americans: A biopsychosocial model. *American Psychologist*. 54: 805–816.

Claudio, L. 1996. New efforts to address childhood asthma in the Bronx. *Environmental Health Perspectives* 104: 1028–1029.

Claudio, L. 2000. Reaching out to New York neighborhoods. *Environmental Health Perspectives* 108: 10.

Claudio, L., L. Tulton, J. Doucette, and P. J. Landrigan. 1999. Socioeconomic factors and asthma hospitalization rates in New York City. *Journal of Asthma* 36: 343–350.

Cohen, L. 2000. Personal communication.

Cole, L., and S. Foster. 2000. *From the ground up: Environmental racism and the rise of the environmental justice movement*. New York: NYU Press.

Collin, R. W., and R. M. Collin. 1998. The role of communities in environmental decisions: Communities speaking for themselves. *Journal of Environmental Law and Litigation*, 13: 37, 39.

Collins, P. H. 1990. *Black feminist thought: Knowledge, consciousness, and the politics of empowerment*. Boston: Unwin Hyman.

Commoner, B. 1992. *Making peace with the planet*. New York: The New Press.

Community Environmental Health Center. 1989. Hazardous neighbors? Living next door to industry in Greenpoint/Williamsburg. New York: Hunter College.

Cooper, M. 1995. Monitoring the north Brooklyn muck: Watchdog steps in. *New York Times*, July 2, CY12.

Corbin-Mark, C. 2001. Program Director, West Harlem Environmental Action. Personal communication.

Council on Environmental Quality. 1996. Considering cumulative effects under the National Environmental Policy Act. Final draft, interagency review version, September 24. Washington, DC.

Cozzens, S. E., and E. J. Woodhouse. 1995. Science, government, and the politics of knowledge. In *Handbook of Science and Technology Studies*, ed. S. Jasanoff et al., 533–553. Thousand Oaks, CA: Sage.

Craig, W. J., and S. Elwood. 1998. How and why community groups use maps and geographic information. *Cartography and Geographic Information Systems* 25 (2): 95–104.

Crain, E. F., K. B. Weiss, P. E. Bijur, M. Hersh, L. Westbrook, and R. E. Stein. 1994. An estimate of the prevalence of asthma and wheezing among inner-city children. *Pediatrics* 94: 356–362.

Crocetti, A. 1994. *WABBA v Guliani*, Affidavit, NY State Supreme Court. Index No. 94/106235.

Daniels, N., B. Kennedy, and I. Kawachi. 2000. *Is inequality bad for our health?* Boston: Beacon Press.

Deegan, M. J. 1990. *Jane Addams and the men of the Chicago School, 1892–1918*. New Brunswick, NJ: Transaction Books.

de Guchteneire, P., I. Krukkert, and G. von Liebenstein. 1999. Best practices on indigenous knowledge. UNESCO's Management of Social Transformations Programme (MOST) and the Centre for International Research and Advisory Networks (CIRAN). The Hague: Netherlands Organization for International Coperation in Higher Education.

De Palo, V. A., P. H. Mayo, P. Friedman, and M. J. Rosen. 1994. Demographic influences on asthma hospital admission rates in New York City. *Chest* 106: 447–451.

Delfino, R. J. 2002. Epidemiological evidence for asthma and exposure to air toxics: Linkages between occupational, indoor, and community air pollution research. *Environmental Health Perspectives* 110 (suppl 4): 573–589.

Derthick, M., ed. 1999. *Dilemmas of scale in America's federal democracy.* Cambridge: Cambridge University Press.

Dewey, J. 1944. *Democracy and education: An introduction to the philosophy of education.* New York: The Free Press.

Dewey, J. 1954. *The public and its problems.* Chicago: Gateway Books.

Diez-Roux, A. 1998. Bringing context back into epidemiology: Variables and fallacies in multilevel analysis. *American Journal of Public Health* 88: 216–22.

Dimaggio, P. J., and W. Powell, eds. 1991. *The new institutionalism in organizational analysis.* University of Chicago Press.

Di Chiro, G. 1998. Environmental justice from the grassroots. In *The Struggle for Ecological Democracy*, ed. Daniel Faber, 104–136. New York: Guilford Press.

Douglas, M., and A. Wildavsky. 1982. *Risk and culture: An essay on the selection of technical and environmental dangers.* Berkeley: University of California Press.

Dowie, M. 1995. *Losing ground: American environmentalism at the close of the twentieth century.* Cambridge, MA: The MIT Press.

Dryzek, J. 1990. *Discursive democracy: Politics, policy, and political science.* Cambridge: Cambridge University Press.

Dryzek, J. 1997. *The politics of the earth: Environmental discourses.* Oxford: Oxford University Press.

Dube, J. 1994. The clouds of dust, not joy: Nabes fight blast cleaning. *Daily News*, September 13.

Du Bois, W. E. B. 1990. *The souls of black folk.* New York: Vintage Books. (Orig. pub. 1903.)

Dubos, R. 1959. *Mirage of health: Utopias, progress, and biological change.* New York: Harper & Row.

Duffy, J. 1990. *The sanitarians: A history of American public health.* Urbana: University of Illinois Press.

Dyson, M. 1993. *Reflecting black: African American cultural criticism.* Minneapolis: University of Minnesota Press.

Eggleston, P. A. 1999. The environment and asthma in U.S. inner cities. *Environmental Health Perspectives*, 104 (7, suppl. 3): 439–450.

Eggleston, P. A., and R. K. Bush. 1999. Environmental allergen avoidance: An overview. *Journal of Allergy and Clinical Immunology* 103: 179–191.

Ehrmann, J. R., and B. L. Stinson. 1999. Joint fact-finding and the use of technical experts. In *The Consensus Building Handbook*, Susskind et al. Thousand Oaks, CA: Sage.

El Puente youth involvement in community health and environment. 2000. Available at http://www.ciet.org/www/image/country/_new-frames.html.

El Puente-CIET household survey on air pollution and health conducted in December, 1995: Some preliminary results. 1995. Draft report. Unpublished data on file with El Puente, Brooklyn, NY.

Emirbayer, M. 1997. Manifesto for a relational sociology. *American Journal of Sociology* 102 (2): 28–17.

Epstein, B. 2000. Personal communication. Health and Environmental Justice Program Coordinator, The Point Community Development Corporation, Hunts Point, the Bronx.

Epstein, S. 1996. *Impure science: AIDS, activism, and the politics of knowledge.* Berkeley: University of California Press.

Ernst, P., K. Demissie, L. Joseph, U. Locher, and M. R. Becklake. 1995. Socio-economic status and indicators of asthma in children. *American Journal Respiratory Critical Care Medicine* 152: 570–575.

Escobar, A. 1997. *Encountering development: The making and unmaking of the Third World.* Princeton, NJ: Princeton University Press

Escobar, A. 1999. After nature: Steps to an antiessentialist political ecology. *Current Anthropology* 40 (1): 1–30.

Evans, R. G., M. L. Marer, and T. R. Marmor. 1994. *Why are some people healthy and others not? The determinants of health of populations.* New York: Aldine de Gruyter.

Ezrahi, Y. 1990. *The descent of Icarus.* Cambridge, MA: Harvard University Press.

Faber, D. 1998. *The struggle for ecological democracy.* New York: Guilford.

Fals Borda, O., and M. A. Rahman, eds. 1991. *Action and knowledge: Breaking the monopoly with participatory action research.* New York: Apex Press.

Farmer, P. 1999. *Infections and inequalities.* Cambridge, MA: Harvard University Press.

Finkel, A., and D. Golding, eds. 1994. Worst things first? The debate over risk-based national environmental priorities. Washington, DC: Resources for the Future.

Fiorino, D. 1989. Environmental risk and democratic process: A critical review. *Columbia Journal of Environmental Law* 14: 501–547.

Fiorino, D. 1990. Citizen participation and environmental risk: A summary of institutional mechanisms. *Science, Technology, and Human Values* 15 (2): 226–244.

Fischer, F. 2000. *Citizens, experts, and the environment: The politics of local knowledge.* Durham, NC: Duke University Press.

Fischer, F., and J. Forester, eds. 1993. *The argumentative turn in policy analysis and planning.* Durham, NC: Duke University Press.

Fitzpatrick, K., and LaGory, M. 2000. *Unhealthy places: The ecology of risk in the urban landscape*. London: Routledge.

Fleming, J. 1999, 2000, 2001. Personal communication.

Forester, J., ed. 1985. *Critical theory and public life*. Cambridge, MA: The MIT Press.

Forester, J. 1989. *Planning in the face of power*. Berkeley: University of California Press.

Forester, J. 1993. Understanding planning practice. In *Critical theory, public policy, and planning practice: Toward a critical pragmatism*. Albany: SUNY Press.

Forester, J. 1999. *The deliberative practitioner*. Cambridge, MA: The MIT Press.

Foucault, M. 1977. *Discipline and punish: The birth of the prison*. New York: Vintage Books.

Foucault, M. 1986. Disciplinary power and subjection. In *Power*, ed. S. Lukes, 229–242. Oxford: Basil Blackwell.

Frankel, S., ed. 1992. *The community health worker: Effective programs for developing countries*. Oxford: Oxford University.

Franzini, L., J. C. Ribble, and A. M. Keddie. 2001. Understanding the Hispanic paradox. *Ethnicity and Disease* 11 (3): 496–518.

Fraser, N., and S. Bartky, eds. 1992. *Revaluing French feminism: Critical essays on difference, agency, and culture*. Bloomington: Indiana University Press.

Freire, P. 1972. *Cultural action for freedom*. Harmondsworth, Middlesex, UK: Penguin.

Freire, P. 1974. *Pedagogy of the oppressed*. New York: The Seabury Press.

Freudenberg, N. 1984. *Not in our backyards: Community action for health and the environment*. New York: Monthly Review Press.

Friedmann, J. 1987. *Planning in the public domain: From knowledge to action*. Princeton, NJ: Princeton.

Funtowicz, S., and J. R. Ravetz. 1993. Science for the post-normal age. *Futures* 25 (7): 739–759.

Funtowicz, S., and J. R. Ravetz. 1999. Post-normal science: An insight now maturing. *Futures* 31: 641–646.

Fullilove, M. 2004. *Root shock: How tearing up city neighborhoods hurts America, and what we can do about it*. New York: Ballantine Press.

Gamson, W. 1992. *Talking politics*. New York: Cambridge University Press.

Garden-Acosta, L. 1999, 2000, 2001, 2002. Personal communication.

Gaventa, J. 1993. The powerful, the powerless, and the experts: Knowledge struggles in an information age. In *Voices of change: Participatory research in the U.S. and Canada*, ed. P. Park, M. Brydon-Miller, B.L. Hall, and T. Jackson, 21–40. Westport, CT: Bergin and Garvey.

Geertz, C. 1983. *Local knowledge: Further essays in interpretive anthropology*. New York: Basic Books.

Geertz, C. 1973. *The interpretation of cultures.* New York: Basic.

Geiger, J. 1967. The neighborhood health center: Education of the faculty in preventative medicine. *Archives of Environmental Health* 14 (6): 912–916.

George, T. 1996. Parents push DOT for lead testing. *New York Daily News,* February 21, p. 1.

Gergen, P. J., and K. B. Weiss. 1995. Epidemiology of asthma. In *Asthma and Rhinitis,* ed. W. W. Busse and S. H. Holgate, 15–31. Boston: Blackwell.

Gergen, P. J., K. M. Mortimer, P. A. Eggleston, D. Rosenstreich, H. Mitchell, D. Ownby, M. Kattan, D. Baker, E. C. Wright, R. Slavin, and F. Malveaux. 1999. Results of the NCICAS environmental intervention to reduce cockroach allergen exposure in inner-city homes. *Journal of Allergy Clinical Immunology* 103 (3, pt 1): 501–506.

Geronimus A. T. 2000. To mitigate, resist, or undo: Addressing structural influences on the health of urban populations. *American Journal of Public Health* 90: 867–872.

Gibbons, M. 1999. Science's new social contract with society. *Nature* 402: C81–84.

Gibbs, L. 1994. Risk assessment from a community perspective. *Environmental Impact Assessment Review* 14 (5/6): 327–335.

Giddens, A. 1984. *The constitution of society.* Cambridge: Polity Press.

Gieryn, T. F. 1995. The boundaries of science. In *Handbook of Science and Technology Studies,* ed. S. Jasanoff et al., 393–443 Thousand Oaks, CA: Sage Publications.

Goffman, E. 1959. *The presentation of self in everyday life.* Garden City, NY: Doubleday.

Goffman, E. 1971. *Relations in public: Microstudies of the public order.* New York: Basic.

Goldman, B. A. 2000. An environmental justice paradigm for risk assessment. *Human and Ecological Risk Assessment* 6 (4): 541–548.

Gonzalez, D. 1995. A bridge from hope to social action. *New York Times,* May 23, A1, B4.

Gottlieb, R. 1993. *Forcing the spring: The transformation of the American environmental movement.* Washington, DC: Island Press.

Graham, J. D., and J. B. Wiener. 1995. Confronting risk tradeoffs. In *Risk vs. risk: Tradeoffs in protecting health and the environment,* ed. J. D. Graham and J. B. Wiener, 1–41. Cambridge, MA: Harvard University Press.

Granovetter, M. 1973. The strength of weak ties. *American Journal of Sociology* 81: 1287–1303.

Greed, C. 1994. The place of ethnography in planning: Or is it "real" research? *Planning Practice and Research* 9 (2): 119–128.

Green, M. 1998. Lead and Kids: Why are 30,000 NYC Children Contaminated? A Report of the NYC Public Advocate Office for the City of New York, February 2.

Greider, K. 1993 Against all odds. *City Limits* (August/September): 34–37.

Grenier, L. 1998. *Working with indigenous knowledge: A guide for researchers.* Ottawa: International Development Research Centre.

Gumperz, J. J. 1982. Ethnic style in political rhetoric. In *Discourse strategies*, ed. J. J. Gumperz. Cambridge: Cambridge.

Guinier, L. 1994. *The tyranny of the majority: Fundamental fairness in representative democracy.* New York: Free Press.

Habermas, J. 1970. Technology and science as "Ideology." In *Toward a Rational Society: Student Protest, Science, and Politics*, 81–127. Boston: Beacon Press.

Habermas, J. 1984. *The theory of communicative action, vol. 1.* Cambridge: Polity Press.

Habermas, J. 1990. *On the logic of the social sciences.* Cambridge: Polity Press.

Hall, P. 1994. *Cities of Tomorrow.* Updated ed. London: Blackwell Publishers.

Hamilton, A. 1943. *Exploring the dangerous trades: The autobiography of Alice Hamilton, M.D.* Boston: Little, Brown.

Hamilton, C. 1994. Concerned citizens of South Central Los Angeles. In *Unequal Protection*, ed. R. Bullard. San Francisco: Sierra Club Books.

Hanhardt, E. 1999, 2000. Director of the Environmental Benefits Program, NYC Department of Environmental Protection. Personal communication.

Haraway D. J. 1991. Situated knowledges: The science question in feminism and the privilege of partial perspective. In *Simians, cyborgs, and women: The reinvention of nature*, ed. D. J. Haraway, 183–201. New York: Routledge.

Harding, S. G. 1991. *Whose science? Whose knowledge?: Thinking from women's lives.* Ithaca, NY: Cornell University Press.

Harley, J. B. 1989. Deconstructing the map. *Cartographica* 26 (2): 1–20.

Harr, J. 1996. *A civil action.* Westminster, MD: Random House.

Harvey, D. 1996. *Justice, nature, and the geography of difference.* Oxford: Blackwell.

Hayden, D. 1995. *The power of place: Urban landscapes as public history.* Cambridge, MA: The MIT Press.

Healey, P. 1997. *Collaborative planning: Shaping places in a fragmented society.* London: Macmillian.

Healey, P. 1999. Insitutionalist analysis, communicative planning, and shaping places. *Journal Planning Education and Research* 19: 111–121.

Hegner, R. 2000. The asthma epidemic: Prospects for controlling an escalating public health crisis. Washington, DC: National Health Policy Forum.

Hesperian Foundation. 1998. Women's health exchange—Reducing workplace health hazards guide: Making a risk map. Berkeley, CA: Hesperian Foundation.

Hevesi, D. 1993. State approves the Brooklyn Navy Yard incinerator; Long-sought permits anger opponents. *New York Times,* Sept. 12, sec. 1, 47(L).

Hevesi, D. 1994. Hasidic and Hispanic residents in Williamsburg try to forge a new unity. *New York Times*, September 18, B47.

Higgins D. L., and M. Metzler. 2001. Implementing community-based participatory research centers in diverse urban settings. *Journal of Urban Health* 78 (3): 488–494.

Hill, M. N., L. R. Bone, and A. M. Butz. 1996. Enhancing the role of community-health workers in research. *Image the Journal of Nursing Scholarship* 28 (3): 221–226.

Hobart, M., ed. 1993. *An anthropological critique of development: The growth of ignorance*. London: Routledge.

Hoch, C. 1994. *What planners do: Power, politics, and persuasion*. Chicago: American Planning Association.

Hofrichter, R. 1993. *Toxic struggles: The theory and practice of environmental justice*. Philadelphia, PA: New Society Publishers.

Holgate, S. T., J. M. Samet, H. S. Koren, and R. L. Maynard, eds. 1999. *Air pollution and health*. San Diego, CA: Academic Press.

Holland, D. F., and G. S. J. Perrott. 1938. Health of the Negro. Part I. Disabling illness among Negroes and low-income White families in New York City—A report of a sickness survey in the spring of 1933. *Milbank Memorial Fund Quarterly* 16: 5–38.

Hollister, R. M., B. M. Kramer, and S. S. Bellin, eds. 1974. *Neighborhood health centers*. Lexington, MA: D.C. Heath and Company.

Holloway, L. 1994. Lawsuit challenges rules on lead. *New York Times*, March 20, sec. 13, p. 10, column 1.

Horton, A. I. 1971. *The Highlander Folk School: A history of its major programs, 1932–1961*. New York: Carlson.

Horton, M. 1998. *The long haul: An autobiography*. New York: Teachers College Press.

Hull House Maps and Papers. 1895. New York: Crowell and Co.

Hymes, D. 1974. *Foundations in sociolinguistics: An ethnographic approach*. Philadelphia: University of Pennsylvania.

Iglesias-Garden, Cecilia. 2000, 2001. Personal communication.

Innes, J. E. 1995. Planning theory's emerging paradigm: Communicative action and interactive practice. *Journal of Planning Education and Research* 14 (3): 183–190.

Innes, J. E. 1996. Planning through consensus building: A new view of the comprehensive planning ideal. *Journal of the American Planning Association* 62 (4): 460–472.

Institute of Medicine (IOM). 1999. *Toward environmental justice: Research, education, and health policy needs*. Washington, DC: National Academy Press.

Institute of Medicine (IOM). 2000. *Clearing the air: Asthma and indoor air exposures*. 2000. Washington, DC: National Academy Press.

International Council for Local Environmental Initiatives (ICLEI). 1993. Community-based environmental management: Greenpoint/Williamsburg Environmental Benefits Program. Toronto: ICLEI.

Irwin, A. 1995. *Citizen science: A study of people, expertise, and sustainable development*. London: Routledge.

Irwin, A. 2001. *Sociology and the environment: A critical introduction to society, nature, and knowledge,* Cambridge: Polity Press.

Israel, B. A., A. J. Schulz, E. A. Parker, and A. B. Becker. 1998. Review of community-based research: Assessing partnership approaches to improve public health. *Annual Review of Public Health* 19: 173–202.

Jablonski, R. 2000. Personal communication. March 22, 2000.

Jackson, R. J., and C. Kochtitzky. 2000. Creating a healthy environment: The impact of the built environment on public health. Sprawl Watch Clearinghouse Monograph Series. Washington, DC: Sprawl Watch Clearing House.

Jasanoff, S. 1985. Peer review in the regulatory process. *Science, technology, and Human Values* 10 (52): 20–32.

Jasanoff, S. 1987. Contested boundaries in policy-relevant science. *Social Studies of Science* 17: 195–230.

Jasanoff, S. 1990. *The fifth branch: Science advisors as policy makers*. Cambridge, MA: Harvard University Press.

Jasanoff, S. 1991. Acceptable evidence in a pluralistic society. In *Acceptable Evidence: Science and Values in Hazard Management*, ed. R. Hollander and D. Mayo, 29–47. New York: Oxford University Press.

Jasanoff, S. 1996. Beyond epistemology: Relativism and engagement in the politics of science. *Social Studies of Science* 26 (2): 393–418.

Jasanoff, S. 1999. The songliness of risk. *Environmental Values* 8 (2): 135–152.

Jasanoff, S., and B. Wynne. 1998. Science and decision making. In *Human choice and climate change*, ed. S. Rayner and E. Malone, 1–87. Columbus: Battelle Press.

Jenkins-Smith, H., and P. Sabatier, eds. 1997. *Policy change and learning: Advocacy coalition approach*. Boulder, CO: Westview.

Johannsen, A. 1992. Applied anthropology and post-modernist ethnography. *Human Organization* 57: 71–81.

Kaminsky, M., S. Klitzman, D. Michaels, and L. Stenvenson. 1992. Health profile of cancer, birth defects, asthma, and childhood lead poisoning in Greenpoint/Williamsburg, first report, December. New York: New York City Department of Health.

Kaminsky, M., S. Klitzman, D. Michaels, and L. Stenvenson. 1993. Health profile of cancer, birth defects, asthma, and childhood lead poisoning in Greenpoint/Williamsburg, second report, June. New York: New York City

Department of Health and CUNY Medical School Department of Community Health and Social Medicine.

Kaminstein, D. S. 1996. Persuasion in a toxic community: Rhetorical aspects of public meetings. *Human Organization* 55 (4): 458–464.

Kammen, D., and D. Hassenzahl. 1999. *Should we risk it? Exploring environmental, health, and technological problem solving*. Princeton, NJ: Princeton University Press.

Kaplan, M. 1969. Advocacy for the poor. *Journal of the American Institute of Planners* 35 (2): 96–101.

Kass, D. 1999, 2000, 2001, 2002. Personal communication.

Kazin, M. 1995. *The populist persuasion: An american history*. New York: Basic Books.

Keller, P., and M. Keller. 1993. *Visual cues: Practical data visualization*. Los Alanitis, CA: IEEE Computer Society Press.

Kellogg Foundation. 2003. Home Grown. Community-University Partnerships. Available at http://www.wkkf/Knowledgebase/Pubs.

Kemp, R. 1985. Planning, public hearings, and the politics of discourse. In *Critical Theory and Public Life,* ed. J. Forester, 177–201. Cambridge, MA: The MIT Press.

Ketas, J. 1999. Personal communication. Assistant Commissioner, New York City Department of Environmental Protection.

King G. 1996. Institutional racism and the medical/health complex: A conceptual analysis. *Ethnic Disease* 6: 30–46.

Kingdon, J. 1984. *Agendas, alternatives, and public policies*. New York: Harper Collins Publishers.

Kinney, P. L., M. Aggarwal, M. E. Northridge, N. A. Janssen, and P. Shepard. 2000. Airborne concentrations of PM(2.5) and diesel exhaust particles on Harlem sidewalks: A community-based pilot study. *Environmental Health Perspec*tives 108: 213–218.

Kochman, R. 1981. *Black and white styles in conflict*. Chicago: University of Chicago.

Kolb, D. 1984. *Experiential learning: Experience as the source of learning and development*. Englewood Cliffs, NJ: Prentice Hall.

Kotler, M. 1969. *Neighborhood government: The local foundations of political life*. New York: Bobbs-Merrill.

Kozol, J. 1995. *Amazing grace: The lives of children and the conscience of a nation*. New York: Crown Publishers.

Kranzler, G. 1995. *Hasidic Williamsburg: A contemporary American Hasidic community*. Northvake, NY: Aronson, Inc.

Krieger, N. 1999. Embodying inequality: A review of concepts, measures, and methods for studying health consequences of discrimination. *International Journal of Health Services* 29: 295–352.

Krieger, N. 2000. Discrimination and health. In *Social epidemiology*, ed. L. Berkman and I. Kawachi, 36–75. New York: Oxford University Press.

Krieger, N. 2001. Theories for social epidemiology in the 21st Century: An ecosocial perspective. *International Journal of Epidemiology* 30: 668–677.

Krieger, N., and E. Fee. 1996. Measuring social inequalities in health in the United States: a review, 1900–1950. *International Journal of Health Services* 26: 391–418.

Krieger, N., Williams, D. R., and Moss, N. E. 1997. Measuring social class in U.S. public health research: Concepts, methodologies, and guidelines. *Annual Review of Public Health* 18: 341–378.

Krimsky, S. 1984. Epistemic considerations on the values of folk-wisdom in Science and Technology. *Policy Studies Review* 3 (2): 246–264.

Krimsky, S., and A. Plough. 1988. *Environmental hazards: Communicating risks as a social process.* Dover, MA: Auburn House.

Krumholz, N., and J. Forester. 1990. *Making equity planning work.* Philadelphia, PA: Temple Univ. Press.

Kuehn, R. 1996. The environmental justice implications of quantitative risk assessment. *University of Illinois Law Review* 103–172.

Kuhn, T. 1962. *The structure of scientific revolutions.* Chicago: University of Chicago Press.

Laird, S. A., ed. 2002. *Biodiversity and traditional knowledge: Equitable partnerships in practice.* London: Earthscan Publications.

Lambert, B. 2000. EPA says lead-paint law may increase risks to children. *New York Times*, September 29, B6.

Landrigan, P. J. 2000. Pediatric lead poisoning: Is there a threshold? *Public Health Reports* 115 (6): 530–531.

Lash, J. 1994. Integrating science, values, and democracy through comparative risk assessment. In Worst things first? The debate over risk-based national environmental priorities, eds. A. Finkel and D. Golding, 69–86. Washington, DC: Resources for the Future.

Latour, B. 1979. *Laboratory life: The social construction of scientific facts.* Beverly Hills: CA Sage Publications.

Latour, B. 1988. *Science in action.* Cambridge, MA: Harvard University Press.

Latour, B. 1993. *We have never been modern.* Cambridge, MA: Harvard University Press.

Lawson, C. 2001. Personal communication

Lazarus, R. 1993. Pursuing environmental justice: The distributional effects of environmental protection. *Northwestern University Law Review* 87: 787–857.

Ledogar, R. 2000, 2001a, 2002. Personal communication.

Ledogar, R. 2001b. Inventory of El Puente survey home remedies. Unpublished personal file.

Ledogar, R. J., and N. Andersson. 1993. Impact estimation through sentinel community surveillance: An affordable epidemiological approach. *Third World Planning Review* 15 (3): 263–272.

Ledogar, R. J., L. Garden-Acosta, and A. Penchaszadeh. 1999. Building international public health vision through local community research: the El Puente-CIET partnership. *American Journal of Public Health* 89: 1795–1797.

Ledogar, R. J., C. Iglesias-Garden, A. Miranda, and L. Monasta. 1998. Evidence-based planning by El Puente: A community organization prepares to Promote asthma Mastery in Brooklyn, New York. Unpublished manuscript.

Ledogar, R., A. Penchaszadeh, C. Iglesias-Garden, and L. Garden-Acosta. 2000. Asthma and Latino cultures: Different prevalence reported among groups sharing the same environment. *American Journal of Public Health* 90: 929–935.

Lee, K. N. 1993. *Compass and gyroscope: Integrating science and politics for the Environment.* Washington, DC: Island Press.

Leikauf, G. D. 2002. Hazardous air pollutants and asthma. *Environmental Health Perspectives* 110 (suppl 4): 505–526.

Levi-Strauss, C. 1962. *The savage mind.* Chicago: University of Chicago Press.

Liff, B. 1999. Bridge's lead paint faces a new attack. *New York Daily News*, August 5, P. 7.

Liff, B. 2000. Waste-transfer permit yanked: Ruling is another victory for Red Hook in trash war. *Daily News*, May 12.

Liff, S. 1992. State OKs City's solid waste plan. *Newsday*, October 29, p. 128.

Lindblom, C. E. 1979. The science of muddling through. *Public Administation Review* 19 (1): 79–88.

Lindblom, C. E., and D. K. Cohen. 1979. *Usable knowledge: Social science and social problem solving.* New Haven, CT: Yale University Press.

Link, B. G., M. E. Northridge, J. C. Phelan, and M. L. Ganz. 1998. Social epidemiology and the fundamental cause concept: On the structuring of effective cancer screens by socioeconomic status. *Milbank Quarterly* 76: 375–402.

Lipsky, M. 1976. *Street-level bureaucracy: Dilemmas of the individual in public services.* New York: Russell Sage Foundation.

Loh, P., and J. Sugerman-Brozan. 2002. Environmental justice organizing for environmental health: Case study on asthma and diesel exhaust in Roxbury, Massachusetts. *Annals of the American Academy of Political and Social Science* 584: 110–124.

Love, M. B., and K. Gardner. 1997. Community health workers: Who they are and what they do? *Health Education and Behavior* 24 (4): 510–522.

Lowi, T. 1969. *The end of liberalism.* New York: W.W. Norton.

Lowry, K., P. Adler, and N. Milner. 1997. Participating the public: Group process, politics, and planning. *Journal of Planning Education and Research* 16 (3): 177–187.

Lynch, K. 1960. *Image of the city*. Cambridge, MA: The MIT Press.

Lynch, M., and S. Woolgar, eds. 1990. *Representation in scientific practice*. Cambridge: The MIT Press.

MacIntyre, S., S. MacIver, and A. Sooman. 1993. Area, class, and health: Should we be focusing on people or places? *Journal of Social Policy* 22: 213–234.

Macintyre, S., A. Ellaway, and S. Cummins,. 2002. Place effects on health: How can we conceptualise, operationalise, and measure them? *Social Science and Medicine* 55 (1): 125–39.

Majone, G. 1989. *Evidence, argument, and persuasion in the policy process*. New Haven, CT: Yale Press.

Mandelbaum, S. 1991. Telling stories. *Journal of Planning Education and Research* 10 (3): 209–214.

Mansbridge, J. 1986. *Why we lost the ERA*. Chicago: University of Chicago Press.

Markides, K. S., and J. Coreil. 1986. The health of Hispanics in the southwestern United States: An epidemiologic paradox. *Public Health Reports* 101 (3): 253–265.

Martin, D. 1998a. Trash station proposal greeted by protest. *New York Times*, March 4.

Martin, D. 1998b. Boroughs battle over trash as last landfill nears close. *New York Times*, Nov. 16, sec. B; p. 1, col. 4, metropolitan desk.

Marmot, M. G., and R. G. Wilkinson. 1999. *The social determinants of health*. Oxford: Oxford University Press.

McFadden, R. D. 1992. Survey finds high cancer rate in 2 neighborhoods in Brooklyn. *New York Times*, May 23, A27.

McGowan, K. 1999. Breathing lessons. *City Limits* (September/October).

McIntyre, A. 1971. The survival of political philosophy. *The Listener* 85.

Meckel, R. A. 1990. *Save the babies: American public health reform and the prevention of infant mortality, 1850–1929*. Baltimore, MD: Johns Hopkins University Press.

Medoff, P., and H. Sklar. 1994. *Streets of hope*. Boston: South End Press.

Melendez, M. 2003. *We took the streets: Fighting for Latino rights with the Young Lords*. New York: St. Martin's Press.

Melosi, M. 2000. *The sanitary city*. Baltimore, MD: Johns Hopkins University Press.

Mendoza, F. S., and E. Fuentes-Afflick. Latino children's health and the family-community health promotion model. *Western Journal of Medicine* 170: 85–92.

Merchant, C. 1992. *Radical ecology: The search for a livable world*. New York: Routledge.

Merton, R. K. 1973. The normative structure of science. In *The sociology of science: Theoretical and empirical investigations*, R.K. Merton, 267–278. Chicago: University of Chicago Press.

Miller, B. 2000. *Fat of the land: Garbage of New York—The last two hundred years*. New York: Four Walls Eight Windows Press.

Miller, J. E. 2000. The effects of race/ethnicity and income on early childhood asthma prevalence and health care use. *American Journal of Public Health* 90 (3): 428–430.

Mills, C. W. 1959. *The sociological imagination*. Oxford: Oxford University.

Milton, K. 1996. *Environmentalism and cultural theory: Exploring the role of anthropology in environmental discourse*. London: Routledge.

Minkler, M., ed. 1997. Community organizing and community building for health. New Brunswick, NJ: Rutgers University Press.

Minkler, M. 2000. Using participatory action research to build healthy communities. *Public Health Report*, 115 (2–3, Mar–Jun): 191–197.

Minkler, M., and N. Wallerstein, eds. 2003. *Community based participatory research for health*. San Francisco, CA: Jossey-Bass.

Mitchell, A. 1992a. Alarm on tainted dust near Williamsburg Bridge. *New York Times*, August 22, sec. 1, p. 1, col. 3.

Mitchell, A. 1992b. High lead levels found near 3 East River bridges. *New York Times*, September 2, sec. B, p. 3. col. 1.

Moberg, D. 1999. Brothers and sisters: Greens and Labor: It's a coalition that gives corporate polluters fits. *Sierra Magazine* (Jan/Feb).

Monmonier, M. 1996. *How to lie with maps*. 2nd ed. Chicago: University of Chicago Press.

Mott, L. 1995. The disproportionate impact of environmental health threats on children of color. *Environmental Health Perspectives* 103 (suppl 6): 33–35.

Mujica, J. 1992. Coloring the hazards: Risk maps, research, and education to fight health hazards. *American Journal of Industrial Medicine* 22: 767–770.

Mukerji, C. 1989. *A fragile power: Scientists and the state*. Princeton, NJ: Princeton University Press.

Mulkay, M. 1976. Norms and ideology in science. *Social Science Information* 15: 637–656.

Mumford, L. 1938. *The culture of cities*. New York: HBJ.

Myers, S. L. 1992a. Dinkins to appoint task force on lead threat in soil. *New York Times*, September 3, sec. B, p. 3, col. 2.

Myers, S. L. 1992b. Lead-test results, meant to reassure, do the opposite. *New York Times*, September 6, sec. 1, p. 49, col. 2.

Myers, S. L. 1992c. Study finds soil tainted by lead in a playground. *New York Times*, December 27, sec. 1, p. 33; col. 5.

National Environmental Justice Advisory Council (NEJAC). 2000. A regulatory strategy for siting and operating waste transfer stations: A response to a recurring environmental justice circumstance: The siting of waste transfer stations in low-income communities and communities of color. Waste and Facility Siting Subcommittee, Waste Transfer Station Working Group, U.S. Environmental Protection Agency. EPA 500-R-00-001.

National Environmental Justice Advisory Council (NEJAC). 2001. Environmental justice and community-based health model discussion: A report on the public meeting convened by the National Environmental Justice Advisory Council, May 23–26, 2000. EPA 300-R-01-002.

National Institute of Environmental Health Sciences (NIEHS). 2000. Environmental justice: Partnerships for communication grants. Division of Extramural Research and Training. Available at http://www.niehs.nih.gov/dert/programs/translat/envjust/ej-desc.htm#shepard.

National Institute of Environmental Health Sciences (NIEHS). 2004. Health Disparities research. Available at http://www.niehs.nih.gov/oc/factsheets/disparity/phome.htm.

National Institutes of Health (NIH). 2003. Guidelines for the diagnosis and management of asthma—Update on selected topics. National Asthma Education and Prevention Program. Bethesda, MD: National Institutes of Health, National Heart, Lung, and Blood Institute, NIH Publication No. 02-5074.

National Institutes of Health (NIH). 2004. What are health disparities? Available at http://healthdisparities.nih.gov/whatare.html.

National Research Council (NRC). 1983. *Risk assessment in the federal government: Managing the process*. Committee on the Institutional Means for Assessment of Risks to Public Health. Washington, DC: National Academy Press.

National Research Council (NRC). 1996. *Understanding risk: Informing decisions in a democratic society*. Committee on Risk Characterization. Washington, DC: National Academy Press.

National Research Council (NRC). 1999. Board on Environmental Studies and Toxicology. *Research priorities for airborne particulate Matter II: Evaluating research progress and updating the portfolio*. Washington, DC: National Academy Press.

Nelkin, D. 1975. The political impact of technical expertise. *Social Studies of Science* 5: 35–54.

Nelkin, D. 1984. Science and technology policy and the democratic process. In *Citizen participation in science policy*, ed. Petersen, 18–39. Amherst: University of Massachusetts Press.

Nelkin, D. 1995. *Selling science: How the press covers science and technology*. New York: W.H. Freeman.

New York City Department of Environmental Protection (NYC DEP). 1996. Greenpoint/Williamsburg Environmental Benefits Program (brochure). Community Environmental Development Group. Corona, NY: NYC DEP.

New York City Department of Environmental Protection (NYC DEP). 1997. Implementing community right-to-know laws in New York City: 1997 annual report. Corona, NY: NYC DEP.

New York City Department of City Planning. 1996. The newest New Yorkers 1990–1994: An analysis of immigration to New York City in the early 1990s.

New York City Department of Health (NYC DOH). 1997. A non-competitive continuation application for NYCDOH provision of 1997–1998 state and community-based childhood lead poisoning prevention program and surveillance of blood lead levels in children. March 24, 1997, #H64/CCH205097-08.

New York City, Department of Health (NYC DOH). 1997. New cases of lead poisoning (at or greater than 20 µg/dl) among children 6 months to 5 years by health districts New York City—1995. Updated 1/23/97.

New York City Department of Health (NYC DOH). 1999. Childhood Asthma Initiative. Available at http://www.nyc.gov/html/doh/html/asthma/ams.html

New York City Department of Health (NYC DOH). 2000. Asthma facts. Community HealthWorks.

New York City, Department of Health (NYC DOH). 2003. Asthma can be controlled. *NYC Vital Signs* 2: 1–4.

New York City Department of Transportation (DOT). 1998. Final environmental impact statement for lead paint removal operations on New York City Department of Transportation bridges. CEQR #96-DOT-005Y. New York: NYC DOT.

New York State Department of Environmental Conservation (DEC). 1988. Order on consent. In the matter of the violations of the New York State Environmental Conservation Law, 17-0801, by the City of New York, Department of Environmental Protection.

New York State Department of Environmental Conservation (DEC). 1996. Chemical residues in fish, bivalves, crustaceans, and a cephalod from the New York–New Jersey Harbor estuary: PCB, organochlorine pesticides, and mercury.

New York State Department of Health (NYS DOH). 1993. New York State dry cleaner survey. Bureau of Toxic Substance Assessment. November. Albany, NY: NYS DOH.

New York State Department of Health (NYS DOH). 1999. Chronic obstructive pulmonay disease and allied conditions—ICD-9 code 493. The Statewide Planning and Research Cooperative System (SPARCS) 1999 annual report. Community District 1—Greenpoint/Williamsburg. Albany, NY: NYS DOH.

Niederman, Rabbi D. 2000, 2001. Personal communication.

Nicolas, S., G. Canada, M. Northridge, B. Ortiz, K. Shoemaker, and B. Jean-Louis. 2003. Asthma in Central Harlem. The Harlem Childrens Zone Asthma Iniative. Unpublished manuscript.

Noble, H. B. 1999. Far more children are hospitalized for asthma, study shows. *New York Times*, July 27, late edition (East Coast), p. B1.

Northridge, M. E. 2001. Personal communication.

Northridge, M., and P. Shepard. 1997. Environmental racism and public health. *American Journal of Public Health* 87: 730–732.

Northridge, M. E., P. L. Kinney, G. L. Chew, P. Shepard, C. Corbin-Mark, and J. Graziano. 2000. Community Outreach and Education Program (COEP) at the NIEHS Center for Environmental Health in northern Manhattan: The basis for conducting scientifically valid, socially relevant research. *Environmental Epidemiology and Toxicology* 2: 142–150.

Northridge, M. E., D. Vallone, C. Merzel, D. Greene, P. Shepard, A. T. Cohall, and C. G. Healton. 2000. The adolescent years: An academic-community partnership in Harlem comes of age. *Journal Public Health Management Practice* 6: 53–60.

Northridge, M. E., J. Yanura, P. L. Kinney, R. M. Santella, P. Shepard, Y. Riojas, M. Aggarwal, and P. Strickland. 1999. Diesel Exhaust exposure among adolescents in Harlem: A community-driven study. *American Journal of Public Health* 89: 998–1002.

O'Brien M. 2000. When harm is not necessary: Risk assessment as diversion. In *Reclaiming the environmental debate: The politics of health in a toxic culture*, ed. R. Hofrichter, 113–134. Cambridge, MA: The MIT Press.

O'Fallon, L. R., and A. Dearry. 2002. Community-based participatory research as a tool to advance environmental health sciences. *Environmental Health Perspectives* 110 (suppl 2): 155–159.

O'Fallon, L. R., G. M. Wolfle, D. Brown, A. Dearry, and K. Olden. 2003. Strategies for setting a national research agenda that is responsive to community needs. *Environmental Health Perspectives* 111: 1855–1860.

O'Neill, J. 1974. *Making sense together: An introduction to wild sociology.* New York: Harper and Row.

O'Neill, M. S. 1996. Helping schoolchildren with asthma breathe easier: Partnerships in community-based environmental health education. *Environmental Health Perspectives* 104: 464–466.

Osleeb, J., D. Kass, H. Blanco, S. R. Zoloth, D. Sivin, and A. Baimonte. 1997. Baseline aggregate environmental loadings (BAEL) profile of Greenpoint/ Williamsburg Brooklyn. New York City Department of Environmental Protection.

Ostro, B., M. Lipsett, J. Mann, H. Braxton-Owens, and M. White. 2001. Air pollution and exacerbation of asthma in African-American children in Los Angeles. *Epidemiology* 12: 200–208.

Ozawa, C. 1991. *Recasting science: Consensual procedures in public policy making.* Boulder, CO: Westview Press.

Ozawa, C. P., and L. E. Susskind. 1985. Mediating science-intensive public policy disputes. *Journal of Policy Analysis and Management* 5 (1): 23–39.

Ozonoff, D., and L. Boden. 1987. Truth and consequences: Health agency responses to environmental health problems. *Science, Technology, and Human Values* 12 (3–4): 70–7.

Park, P. 1993. What is participatory research? A theoretical and methodological perspective. In *Voices of change: Participatory research in the United States and*

Canada, ed. P. Park, M. Brydon-Miller, B. Hall, and T. Jackson, 1–19. Westport, CT: Bergin & Garvey.

Parker, E. A., A. J. Schulz, B. A. Israel, and R. Hollis. 1998. Detroit's East Side Village Health Worker Partnership: Community-based lay health advisor intervention in an urban area. *Health Education and Behavior* 25 (1): 24–45.

Parker, E. A., B. A. Israel, M. Williams, W. Brakefield-Caldwell, T. C. Lewis, T. Robins, E. Ramirez, Z. Rowe, and G. Keeler. 2003. Community action against asthma: Examining the partnership process of a community-based participatory research project. *Journal of General Internal Medicine* 18 (7): 558–567.

Pasher, I. 2000, 2001. Personal communication.

Paustenbach, D. J., ed. 1989. *The risk assessment of environmental and human health hazards.* New York: Wiley and Sons.

Pearce, N. 1996. Traditional epidemiology, modern epidemiology, and public health. *American Journal of Public Health* 86: 678–683.

Pearce, N., J. Douwes, and R. Beasley. 2000. Is allergen exposure the major primary cause of asthma? *Thorax* 55: 424–431.

Pearce, N., R. Beasley, C. Burgess, and J. Crane. 1998. *Asthma epidemiology: Principles and methods.* New York: Oxford University Press.

Peattie, L. R. 1968. Reflections on advocacy planning. *Journal of the American Institute of Planners* 34 (2): 80–88.

Penchaszadeh, A. 1999, 2000, 2001. Director of El Puente's Environmental Health and Justice Programs. Personal communication.

Perris, R., and J. Chait. 1998. Williamsburg waterfront 197-a plan, A matter of balance: Housing, industry, open space in community board 1. The Municipal Art Society Planning Center, Pratt Institute Center for Community and Environmental Development, Brooklyn, NY.

Pew Environmental Health Commission (Pew). 2000. Attack asthma: Why America needs a public health defense system to battle environmental threats. Baltimore, MD: Johns Hopkins School of Public Health.

Pickering, A., ed. 1992. *Science as practice and culture.* Chicago: Chicago University Press.

Piore, M. J. 1995. *Beyond individualism.* Cambridge, MA: Harvard University Press.

Piven, F. F., and R. Cloward. 1979. *Poor people's movements: Why they succeed, How they fail.* New York: Vintage.

Platts-Mills, T., ed., 1999. *Asthma: Causes and mechanisms of an epidemic inflammatory disease.* New York: Lewis Publishers.

Plough, A., and S. Krimsky. 1988. *Environmental hazards: Communicating risks as a social process.* Westport, CT: Auburn House

Polanyi, M. 1962. The Republic of Science. *Minerva.* 1: 54–73.

Porter, D. 1997. *Social medicine and medical sociology in the twentieth century.* Amsterdam: Rodopi Books.

Porter, T. 1995. *Trust in numbers.* Princeton, NJ: Princeton University Press.

Powell, W. W., and P. J. DiMaggio, eds. 1991. *The new institutionalism in organizational analysis.* Chicago: University of Chicago Press.

Presidential/Congressional Commission on Risk Assessment and Risk Management (PCRARM). 1997. Framework for environmental health risk management.

Pressman, J. L., and A. Wildavsky. 1973. *Implementation.* Berkeley: University of California Press.

Price, D. K. 1965. *The scientific estate.* Cambridge, MA: Harvard University Press.

Putnam, H. 1992. A reconsideration of Deweyan democracy. In *Renewing philosophy,* ed. H. Putnam. Cambridge, MA: Harvard University Press.

Putnam, H. 1995. *Pragmatism: An open question.* Cambridge, MA: Blackwell.

Putnam, R. 1993. *Making democracy work: Civic traditions in modern Italy.* Princeton, NJ: Princeton University Press.

Quackenboss, J. J., M. Krzyzanowski, and M. D. Lebowitz. 1991. Exposure assessment approaches to evaluate respiratory health effects of particulate matter and nitrogen dioxide. *Journal of Exposure, Analysis, and Environmental Epidemiology* 1: 83–107.

Raffensperger, C., and J. Tickner. 1999. *Protecting public health and the environment: Implementing the precautionary principle.* Washington, DC: Island Press.

Raiffa, H. 1982. *The art and science of negotiation.* Cambridge, MA: Harvard University Press.

Ramirez-Valles, J. 1998. Promoting health, promoting women: The construction of female and professional identities in the discourse of community health workers. *Social Science and Medicine* 47 (11): 1749–1762.

Rao, M., R. E. Kravath, D. Abadco, and P. Steiner. 1991. Childhood asthma mortality: The Brooklyn experience and a brief review. *Journal of the Association for Academic Minority Physicians* 2 (3): 127–130.

Ravetz, J. 1999. What is post-normal science? *Futures* 31: 647–654.

Rawls, J. 1997. The idea of public reason revisited. *University of Chicago Law Review* 64 (3): 765–807.

Reich, R. B. 1988. Policymaking in a democracy. In *The Power of Public Ideas,* ed. R. B. Reich. Cambridge, MA: Harvard University Press.

Reich, R. B. 1991. *The work of nations: Preparing ourselves for 21st century capitalism.* New York: Alfred A. Knopf.

Rein, M. 1969. Social planning: The search for legitimacy. *Journal of the American Institute of Planners* 35 (4): 233–244.

Rein, M. 1983. *From policy to practice.* Armonk, NY: M.E. Sharpe, Inc.

Rein, M., and D. A. Schön. 1980. Problem setting in policy research. *Using social research in public policy making*, ed. Carol Weiss. New York: Columbia University Press.

Rios et al. 1993. Susceptibility to environmental pollutants among minorities. *Toxicology and Industrial Health* 797: 798–803.

Roberts, S. M. 2000: Environmental justice: Examining the role of risk assessment. *Human and Ecological Risk Assessment* 6 (4): 537–540.

Robbins, P. 2003. Beyond ground truth: GIS and the environmental knowledge of herders, professional foresters, and other traditional communities. *Human Ecology* 31 (2): 233–239.

Rodriguez, N. 1999. Personal communication.

Rose, F. 2000. *Coalitions across the class divide*. Ithaca, NY: Cornell University Press.

Rosen, G. 1985. The first neighborhood health center movement. In *Sickness and Health in America*, eds. J. W. Leavitt and R. L. Numbers, 475–489. University of Wisconsin Press.

Rosen, G. 1993. *A history of public health*. Expanded ed. Baltimore, MD: Johns Hopkins University Press.

Rosen, J. 1994. Affidavit February 25. Professor of pediatrics and head of the Division of Environmental Sciences at Albert Einstein College of Medicine and attending physician at Montefiore Medical Center, Bronx, New York. New York State Supreme Court, County of New York. Index No. 94/106235.

Rosenbaum, A. S., D. A. Axelrad, T. J. Woodruff, Y. H. Wei, M. P. Ligocki, and J. P. Cohen. 1999. National estimates of outdoor air toxics concentrations. *Journal of the Air Waste Management Association* 49: 1138–1152.

Rosenberg, C. 1992. Explaining epidemics and other studies in the history of medicine. Cambridge: Cambridge University Press.

Rosenstreich, D., P. Eggleston, M. Kattan, et al. 1997. The role of cockroach allergy and exposure to cockroach allergen in causing morbidity among inner-city children with asthma. *New England Journal of Medicine* 336: 1356–1363

Ruckelshaus, W. D. 1984. Risk in a free society. *Risk Analysis* 4: 157–162.

Ruff, H., M. Markowitz, P. Bijur, and J. Rosen. 1996. Relationships among blood lead levels, iron deficiency, and cognitive development in two-year-old children. *Environmental Health Perspectives* 104: 180–185.

Sabatier, P. A., and H. C. Jenkins-Smith, eds. 1993. *Policy change and learning: An advocacy coalition approach*. Boulder, CO: Westview Press.

Sabel, C., A. Fung, and B. Karkkainen. 1999. Beyond backyard environmentalism: How communities are quietly refashioning environmental regulation. *Boston Review* (Oct/Nov).

Sagoff, M. 1988. *Economy of the earth*. Cambridge: Cambridge University Press.

Saltonstall, D. 1998. Down in the dumps: Greenpoint, Williamsburg fighting against proposed garbage site. *Daily News*, May 17.

Saulny, S., and A. C. Revkin. 2001. E.P.A. says air is safe, but public is doubtful. *New York Times*, sec. B, col. 1; metropolitan desk, p. 9.

Schantz, S. L., D. M. Gasior, E. Polverejan, R. J. McCaffrey, A. M. Sweeney, H. E. Humphrey, and J. C. Gardiner. 2001. Impairments of memory and learning in older adults exposed to polychlorinated biphenyls via consumption of Great Lakes fish. *Environmental Health Perspectives* 109 (6): 605–611.

Schlosberg, D. 1999. *Environmental justice and the new pluralism: The challenge of difference for environmentalism*. Oxford: Oxford University Press.

Schön, D. 1971. *Beyond the stable state*. New York: Random House.

Schön, D. 1983. *The reflective practitioner*. New York: Basic Books.

Schön, D., and M. Rein. 1994. *Frame reflection: Toward the resolution of intractable policy controversies*. New York: Basic Books.

Schorr, L. B., and J. T. English. 1974. Background, context and significant issues in neighborhood health center programs. In *Neighborhood Health Centers*, ed. R. M. Hollister, B. M. Kramer, and S. S. Bellin. Lexington, MA: D.C. Heath and Company.

Schultz, A. J., B. A. Israel, S. M. Selig, I. S. Bayer, and C. B. Griffin. 1998. Development and implementation of principles for community-based research in public health. In *Research strategies for community practice*, ed. R. H. MacNair, 83–110. New York: Haworth Press.

Schutz, A. 1976. *The phenomenology of the social world*, trans. G. Walsh and F. Lehnert. London: Heineman.

Schwartz, J. 1994. Low-level lead exposure and children's IQ: A meta-analysis and search for a threshold. *Environment* 65: 42–55.

Science Advisory Board (SAB) 1999. Integrated environmental decision-making in the twenty-first century. Integrated Risk Project Steering Committee, U.S. Environmental Protection Agency. Available at http://www.epa.gov/sab.1999.

Sclove, R. 1995. *Democracy and technology*. New York: Guilford Press.

Sclove, R. 1996. Town meetings on technology. *Technology Review* 99 (5): 24–31

Scott, J. C. 1998. *Seeing like a state: How certain schemes to improve the human condition have failed*. New Haven, CT: Yale University Press.

Scott, J. C. 1990. *Domination and the arts of resistance*. New Haven, CT: Yale University Press.

Sen, A. 1999. *Development as freedom*. New York: Alfred A. Knopf.

Sexton, J. 1997. In a part of Brooklyn, the new welfare rules change everything. *New York Times*, March 10.

Sexton, J. 1998. Amid anxiety, glimpses of hope: Southside adopts to a new, uncertain world of welfare. *New York Times*, January 4.

Sexton, K. 2000. Socioeconomic and racial disparities in environmental health: Is risk assessment part of the problem or part of the solution? *Human and Ecological Risk Assessment* 6 (4): 561–574.

Shapin, S. 1994. *A social history of truth*, 65–86. Chicago: University of Chicago Press.

Shaw, R. 1996. *The activist's handbook: A primer for the 1990s and beyond.* Berkeley, CA: University of California Press.

Shell, E. R. 2000. Does civilization cause asthma? *Atlantic Monthly* 285:90–100.

Shin, P. H. B. 1999. Waste probe launched: Garbage transfer is tops on fed's list. *Daily News*, March 9, suburban, p. 1.

Shiva, V. 1997. *Biopiracy: The plunder of nature and knowledge.* Boston: South End Press.

Shiva, V. 2000. *Stolen harvest: The hijacking of the global food supply.* Boston: South End Press.

Sicherman, B. 1984. *Alice Hamilton: A life in letters.* Cambridge, MA: Harvard University Press.

Silbergeld, E. K. 1997. Preventing lead poisoning in children. *Annual Review of Public Health* 18:187–210.

Silverman, D. 1993. *Interpreting qualitative data: Methods for analyzing talk, text, and interaction.* London: Sage.

Simon, H. 1976. *Administrative behavior: A study of decision-making processes,* 3d ed. New York: Free Press.

Singer, M. 1994. Community-centered praxis: Toward an alternative non-dominative applied anthropology. *Human Organization* 53 (4): 336–344.

Skocpol, T. 1999. Advocates without members: The recent transformation of American civic life. In *Civic engagement in American democracy*, ed. T. Skocpol and M. P. Fiorina, 461–506. Washington, DC: Brookings.

Sloan, R., B. Young, and K. Harrala. 1995. PCB paradigms for striped bass in New York State. Albany, NY: NYS DEC.

Smith, K., C. B. Barrett, and P. W. Box. 2000. Participatory risk mapping for targeting research and assistance: With an example from East African pastoralists. *World Development* 28 (11): 1945–1959.

Smitherman, G. 2000. *Talking that talk: Language, culture, and education in African America.* New York: Routledge.

Spirn, A. W. 1984. *The granite garden: Urban nature and human design.* New York: Basic Books.

Steingraber, S. 1998. *Living downstream: A scientist's personal investigation of cancer and the environment.* New York: Vintage Books.

Steinsapir, C., K. Schwarz, and D. Lalor. 1992. Right-to-breathe/right-to-know: Industrial air pollution in Greenpoint-Williamsburg. A special report by the Community Environmental Health Center. New York: Hunter College.

Stolberg, S. 1999. Poor people are fighting baffling surge in asthma. *New York Times*, Oct. 18, A18.

Stone, D. 1988. *Policy paradox and political reason*. New York: Harper Collins Publishers.

Story, M., and L. J. Harris. 1989. Food habits and dietary change of Southeast Asian refugee families living in the United States. *Journal of American Dietary Association* 89: 800–803.

Stout, D. 1996a. Court halts Williamsburg Bridge cleaning in battle over showers of lead paint. *New York Times*, June 22, sec. 1, p. 23, col. 1.

Stout, D. 1996b. Accord reached in suit over East River bridges. *New York Times*, November 16, sec. 1, p. 27, col. 5.

Sullivan, J. 1995. Plan to build incinerator faces delay; Navy Yard project is being postponed. *New York Times*, June 16, B4.

Susser, M., and E. Susser. 1996. Choosing a future for epidemiology I: Eras and paradigms. *American Journal of Public Health* 86: 668–673.

Susskind, L. 1994. *Environmental diplomacy: Negotiating more effective global agreements*. Oxford: Oxford University Press.

Susskind, L., and J. Cruikshank. 1987. *Breaking the impasse: Consensual approaches to resolving public disputes*. New York: Basic Books.

Susskind, L., and M. Elliot. 1983. *Paternalism, conflict, and co-production*. New York: Plenum Publishers.

Susskind, L., R. K. Jain, and A. O. Martyniuk. 2001. *Better environmental policy studies*. Washington, DC: Island Press.

Susskind, L., P. Levy, and J. Thomas-Larmer. 1999. *Negotiating environmental agreements: How to avoid escalating confrontation, needless costs, and unnecessary litigation*. Washington, DC: Island Press.

Susskind, L., S. McKearnen, and J. Thomas-Lamar. 1999. *The consensus building handbook*. New York: Sage.

Swanston S. 1999, 2000, and 2001. Personal communication.

Sweeney, J., C. Shipman, and A. Tassi. 1994. The Environmental Benefits Program, Brooklyn, NY. The Mega Cities Project. Urban environment-poverty case study series. New York: United Nations Development Program.

Sydenstricker, E. 1933. *Health and environment*. New York: McGraw Hill Co.

Szasz, A. 1994. *Ecopopulism: Toxic waste and the movement for environmental justice*. Minneapolis: University of Minnesota Press.

Talcott F. 1999, 2000. Personal communication.

Tauxe, C. S. 1995. Marginalizing public participation in local planning: An ethnographic account. *Journal American Planning Association* 61 (4): 471–481.

Taylor, D. 2000. The rise of the environmental justice paradigm: Injustice framing and the social construction of environmental discourses. *American Behavioral Scientist* 43 (4): 508–581.

Tesh, S. N. 1988. *Hidden arguments: Political ideology and disease prevention policy.* New Brunswick, NJ: Rutgers University Press.

Tesh, S. N. 1996. Miasma and "social factors" in disease causality: Lessons from the nineteenth century. *Journal of Health Politics, Policy, and Law* 20 (4).

Tesh, S. N. 2000. *Uncertain hazards: Environmental activists and scientific proof.* Ithaca, NY: Cornell University Press.

Throgmorton, J. A. 1996. *Planning as persuasive storytelling: The rhetorical construction of Chicago's electric future.* Chicago: University of Chicago Press.

Thrupp, L. 1989. Legitimatizing local knowledge: "Scientized packages" or empowerment for Third World people. In *Indigenous knowledge systems: Implications for agriculture and international development,* ed. D. M. Warren, J. Slikkerveer, and S. O. Titilola, 138–153. Studies in Technology and Social Change No. 11. Ames: Iowa State University, Technology and Social Change Program.

Tribe, L. H. 1972. Policy science: Analysis or ideology? *Philosophy and Public Affairs* 2 (66).

Tushman, M. 1977. Special boundary roles in the innovation process. *Administrative Science Quarterly* 22: 587–605.

Tushman, M., and T. J. Scanlan. 1981. Boundary spanning individuals: Their role in information transfer and their antecedents. *Academy of Management Journal* 24 (2): 289–305.

U.S. Bureau of Census. 2000. Population and income file, Stf3a. Washington, DC: U.S. Department of Commerce. Available at http://www.census.gov/main/www/cen2000.html.

U.S. Department of Health and Human Services (DHHS). 2000. *Healthy people 2010: Understanding and improving health.* 2nd ed. Washington, DC: U.S. Government Printing Office.

U.S. Environmental Protection Agency (US EPA). 1986. Guidelines for carcinogenic risk assessment. *Federal Register* (September 24) 51: 339992–35003.

U.S. Environmental Protection Agency (US EPA). 1992. Reducing risk: Setting priorities and strategies for environmental protection. Washington, DC: U.S. EPA Science Advisory Board.

U.S. Environmental Protection Agency (US EPA). 1993. Fish sampling and analysis. Vol. 1 of Guidance for assessing chemical containment data for use in fish advisories. Office of Water. EPA 832-R-93-002. Washington, DC: U.S. Environmental Protection Agency.

U.S. Environmental Protection Agency (US EPA). 1994. Guidance for conducting fish and wildlife consumption surveys. Office of Water. EPA 823-B-98-007. Washington, DC: U.S. Environmental Protection Agency.

U.S. Environmental Protection Agency (US EPA). 1997. Cumulative risk assessment guidance. Science Policy Council. Available at http://www.epa.gov/ORD/spc/2cumrisk.htm.

U.S. Environmental Protection Agency (US EPA). 1999a. Office of Policy, Planning, and Evaluation. Community-specific cumulative exposure assessment for Greenpoint/Williamsburg, New York. Washington, DC: US EPA.

U.S. Environmental Protection Agency (US EPA). 1999b. Comparative dietary risks: Balancing the risks and benefits of fish consumption. Toxicology excellence for risk assessment, August 6. Washington, DC: US EPA.

U.S. Environmental Protection Agency (US EPA). 2000. The cumulative exposure project. Available at http://www.epa.gov/oppecumm/.

U.S. Environmental Protection Agency (US EPA). 2001. The cumulative exposure project. Available at http://www.epa.gov/cumulativeexposure/.

U.S. Environmental Protection Agency (US EPA). 2004. National Environmental Justice Advisory Committee. Cumulative risk assessment and environmental justice. Draft guidance, March. Washington, DC: US EPA.

Van der Ploeg, J. D. 1993. Potatoes and knowledge. In *An anthropological critique of development: The growth of ignorance*, ed. M. Hobart, 209–227. London: Routledge.

Van Natta, D., Jr. 1995. Judge halts Bridge Effort on lead paint. *New York Times,* October 7, sec. 1, p. 21, col. 5.

Vedal, S., J. Petkau, R. White, and J. Blair. 1998. Acute effects of ambient inhalable particles in asthmatic and nonasthmatic children. *American Journal of Respiratory Critical Care Medicine* 157: 1034–1043.

Waldman, A. 1997. Concern grows on where trash will go after Fresh Kills. *New York Times*, Nov. 16, sec. 14, col. 3.

Wallace, D., E. Groth, E. Kirrane, B. Warren, and J. Halloran. 1995. Upstairs, downstairs: Perchloroethylene in the air in apartments above New York City dry cleaners. October 1995. Yonkers, NY: Consumers Union of the United States, Inc.

Warren, D. M. 1991. Using indigenous knowledge in agricultural development. World Bank Discussion Paper No. 127. Washington, DC: The World Bank.

Warren, D. M., G. W. von Liebenstein, and L. Slikkerveer. 1993. Networking for indigenous knowledge. *Indigenous Knowledge and Development Monitor* 1 (1): 2–4.

Wates, N., ed. 2000. *The community planning handbook*. London: Earthscan.

Watchperson Project. 1999. Maps and unpublished data.

Waterfront Week. 1999. A publication of happenings in the Greenpoint/Williamsburg community. Fishing awareness day, May 1, 1999.

Weinberg, A. M. 1972. Science and trans-science. *Minerva* 10: 209–222.

Wenger, E. 1998. *Communities of practice: Learning, meaning, and identity*. Cambridge: Cambridge University Press.

Werner, D. 1981. The village health worker: Lackey or liberator? *World Health Forum* 2: 46–68.

Wernette, D. R., and L. A. Nieves. 1992. Breathing polluted air. *EPA Journal* 18: 16–17.

West, P., J. M. Fly, R. Marans, F. Larkin, and D. Rosenblatt, 1995. Minorities and toxic fish consumption: Implications for point discharge policy in Michigan. In *Environmental justice: Issues, policies and solutions*, ed. B. Bryant, 124–137. Washington, DC: Island Press.

Whitney, J. S., ed. 1934. Death rates by occupation based on data of the U.S. Census Bureau 1930. New York: National Tuberculosis Association.

Whyte, W., ed. 1991. *Participatory action research*. Newbury Park, CA: Sage.

Whyte, W. F. 1943. *Street corner society*. Chicago: University of Chicago Press.

Wildavsky, A. 1979. *Speaking truth to power: The art and craft of policy analysis*. Boston: Little, Brown.

Wildavsky, A., and L. Levenson. 1995. Do rodent studies predict cancer in human beings? In *But is it true? A citizen's guide to environmental health and safety issues*, ed. A. Wildavsky, 247–273. Cambridge, MA: Harvard University Press.

Williams, D. R., and C. Collins. 1995. U.S. socioeconomic and racial differences in health: Patterns and explanations. *Annual Review of Sociology* 21: 349–386.

Wilson, R., and E. Crouch. 1987. Risk assessment and comparisons: An introduction. *Science* 236: 267–270.

Winner, L. 1986. *The whale and the reactor: A search for limits in an age of high technology*. Chicago: University of Chicago Press.

Witmer, A., S. D. Seifer, L. Finocchio, J. Leslie, and E. H. O'Neill. 1995. Community health workers: Integral members of the health care work force. *American Journal of Public Health* 85: 1055–1058.

Woodruff, T. J., D. A. Axelrad, J. Caldwell, R. Morello-Frosch, and A. Rosenbaum, 1998. Public health implications of 1990 air toxics concentrations across the United States. *Environmental Health Perspectives* 106: 245–251.

Woolcock, A. J., and J. K. Peat. 1997. Evidence for the increase in asthma worldwide. *Ciba Foundation Symposia*, 206: 122–134.

Wolfgang, A., ed. 1979. *Nonverbal behavior: Applications and cultural implications*. New York: Academic.

Wollgar, S. 1988. *Science: The very idea*. London: Routledge.

World Bank. 1999. World development report 1998/1999: Knowledge for development. Available at http://econ.worldbank.org/wdr/.

World Health Organization (WHO). 1997. Indicators for policy and decision making in environmental health, draft. Geneva, Switzerland: WHO.

Wynne, B. 1989. Frameworks of rationality in risk management: Towards the testing of naive sociology. In *Environmental threats: Perception, analysis, and management*, ed. J. Brown, 33–47. London: Belhaven Press.

Wynne, B. 1991. Knowledges in context. *Science, Technology, and Human Values* 16: 111–121.

Wynne, B. 1996. May the sheep graze safely: A reflective view of the expert-lay knowledge divide. In *Risk, environment, and modernity: Towards a new ecology*, ed. S. Lash, 44–83. London: Sage.

Wynne, B. 1996. Misunderstood misunderstandings: Social identities and public uptake of science. In *Misunderstanding science? The public reconstruction of science and technology*, ed. A. Irwin and B. Wynne, 19–46. Cambridge: Cambridge University Press.

Yearley, S. 1994. Understanding science from the perspective of the sociology of scientific knowledge: An overview. *Public Understanding of Science* 3: 245–258.

Yearley, S. 1999. Computer models and the public's understanding of science: A case-study analysis. *Social Studies of Science* 29: 845–866.

Yearley, S. 2000. Making systematic sense of public discontents with expert knowledge: Two analytical approaches and a case study. *Public Understanding of Science* 9: 105–122.

Young, I. 1990. *Justice and the politics of difference*. Princeton, NJ: Princeton University Press.

Young, I. 1996. Communication and the other: Beyond deliberative democracy. In *Democracy and difference*. ed. S. Benhabib. Princeton, NJ: Princeton University Press.

Zahm, S. H., L. M. Pottern, D. R. Lewis, M. H. Ward, and D. W. White. 1994. Inclusion of women and minorities in occupational cancer epidemiologic research. *Journal of Occupational Medicine* 36 (8): 842–847.

Zayas, L., and P. Ozuah. 1996. Mercury use in Espiritismo: A survey of botanicas. *American Journal of Public Health* 86: 111–112.

Index